Single Moms Can Succeed

By

Cathy Wilson

Single Moms Can Succeed

Copyright © 2019

ISBN: 9781698470160

Warning and Disclaimer

Publisher contact

Skinny Bottle Publishing

books@skinnybottle.com

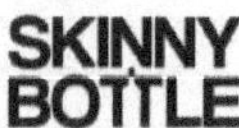

First Words

"Don't ever quit. Right now is difficult, tomorrow might be harder, but the next day the sun will shine brightly." CAW

By using my journey as a single mom to six children, the magical, bad and the downright ugly, I hope to help inspire and open the door to better decision making from other single moms that are struggling to find themselves and provide a positive mindset for their children.

It isn't easy but it's certainly possible.

I want to let other moms know as long as they are doing the best they can, they should be proud of themselves.

I'd like to use my life experiences as a tool to encourage other women to accept and love themselves for doing the best they can. I want to give hope and positively influence you to keep on going no matter how much life kicks the crap out of you.

There's always hope.

There's always tomorrow.

There's always good in everything. Sometimes you've just got to dig deeper.

If I can help just one person feel better then I'm smiling inside out. I yearn to lift women up and help them gain strength through my screw-ups. You deserve to be happy.

Why people look to hurt the already wounded I will never understand.

I am trying to be courageous by opening up, not for sympathy but to use my life journey to help other women any way I can. Hopefully you will screw up less than me. That's the plan anyway.

A few things I'm going to tackle…

1-Talking candidly about the struggles single moms and dads go through in basic.

2-Speaking truthfully through my heart and personal experience even when that leaves me openly vulnerable. Terrified some of the time.

3-Reflect on various challenges with positive take action steps. It's great to acknowledge what is but that's useless unless you know how to challenge the roadblock.

4-Share numerous inspirational quotes I've written that help me push through the tough days and continue to be optimistic even when I only see darkness.

"To be courageous is all about being scared to death…but you choose to hop in the saddle anyway." CAW

Chapter One

A Little About My Family Upbringing

"I essentially had a really happy childhood; most of the scars I bear are self-inflicted."

I could seriously go on forever here but I promise you I'll try and keep it somewhat brief. Before I start I'd like to say that becoming a single parent by choice or not has little to do with your childhood. I'm a perfect example of that.

I'm just opening that door so you can better understand who I am and perhaps why I made some of the life choices I did. Hopefully, it will help me understand more too.

My childhood in a nutshell...

I grew up on a dairy farm with an amazing family. A loving father and mother and three sisters and one brother. We learned early on what hard work was all about and I was lucky we always had everything we needed.

We traveled together on a regular basis and I was involved in many highly competitive sports from basketball and baseball, to volleyball, ringette, and hockey. I was happy and mischievous and loved a challenge. That's what made me a better me. I never stopped until I won, with a smile of course.

I was a tomboy and very close to my father. Out helping him in the barn from the age of two or three. I did well in school and had may friends wherever I went. There was never any major issues in the family other than a little normal squabbling between siblings.

You could say I had no fear growing up. At the age of 2.5, I climbed our 60-foot silo and waved happily from the top to my parents watching from far below. I got lost in the cornfield overnight on our babysitter around the same age and got caught on the power takeoff of the tractor. That broke my arm in 3 places and I was in traction in the hospital for three weeks. Dad told me I wasn't happy to be put back in a crib and diapers while I was in the hospital. But I made it through.

I had long blond hair and chestnut brown eyes with a beautiful bright smile. Apparently, that helped me get away with lots!

My dad was funny and supportive. He taught me to learn by doing and never whine. I see now that it made me a little tougher than I should likely be. Mom was sweet and loving. I'm convinced they got married so she could keep an eye on my dad! Lol! The perfect match in my eyes.

An amazing childhood when I look back. Balanced and loving, strong and morally based. We knew right from wrong and when we challenged things the wrong way we knew there would be a consequence.

Just so you know, I was the one that got spanked the most and frankly I deserved it. My dad did it the right way. When I did something very wrong I got a few swats on the bum and sent it to my room. A few minutes later dad would come up and talk to me about it. Give me a hug and a kiss and he always made sure I know why I got spanked.

Of course, I never liked it at the time but I understand now it was to teach me right from wrong and keep me safe.

My oldest sister was pretty close to me growing up. She was naturally smart and also did well in sports. I just always made sure I was a little bit better. That's the competitive nature coming out in me. The one my father instilled in me and I wouldn't change it for the world.

My first younger sister is Carla. She liked to go against the norm. She did okay in school and liked to play sports too.

My brother was quiet. He helped dad in the barn like we all did, played hockey, did okay in school and put up with all the women in the house! Lol, He has a great judge of character and has strong morals that have proven him well.

My youngest sister is the most like me. She was hugely athletic and did well in school. She's got more of a sound head on her shoulders than me and has lots of great friends for good reason.

We had/have a huge extended family that we were very close to. At least a hundred to our big Christmas and we were always making a point of visiting our cousins on a regular basis. Most of my family was in the agricultural and located fairly close to each other.

We had cottages to go to in the summer and went skiing, snowmobiling, skating, and sledding in the winter. It was tough to find us home on a weekend because we were always away at some sort of sports tournament.

I really couldn't have been luckier growing up.

K- I'm going to stop there because I could write forever on the magic I experienced growing up.

"Family should be the best thing you could ever dream of. They should be there for you during your life highs and lows and love you unconditionally. That's what family is." CAW

Reflection - You don't really have the means to control your childhood. That's when you trust in your mom and dad or parental figure to make the best decisions they can for you. Positive or negative you need to look for the good in your younger years and use that power to make you stronger in the now. I was blessed with an amazing family and for that, I will be forever grateful.

Take Action Steps - There isn't much I would change in my childhood if I could. Except maybe I should have listened more to my dad about become a teacher. That would have helped alleviate the stress I have now of missing my children and not personally having the financial stability I need.

With a stable income and lots of time off I'm sure I would have made different decisions. However, we can't turn back the clocks so onward with a smile.

Chapter Two

Coles Notes Of My Marriage

"Often it's a lack of friendship that makes a marriage unhappy."

Where do I start? Silly asking you I know so I guess I'll just dive right in and I promise to keep it as brief as I can.

After high school, I went to two different universities for degrees, Environmental Studies Geography, and Science of Nutrition. During my second degree, I met my then-husband. It didn't take long for us to decide we wanted to get married. He was a Chinese French Canadian and I was just ready to get married.

Keep in mind I grew up old-fashioned in a sense. In a farm family where you were expected to get your degree, buy your house, find your husband, get married, and start having kids. Not quite like that but that's how I felt.

We didn't have any money, but we got married and figured out a way to make ends meet. I was in restaurant management at the time and he was a sous-chef. Lots of hours but when you are young and energetic, that really doesn't phase you much.

We were living in the city when I finally found out I was expecting my first. We both agreed Toronto was not the place to raise a family so we decided to pick a spot on the map and move north to get established. We wound up at Blue Mountain because my then-husband had a secure sous-chef position at the Pottery dining room, a well-established restaurant at the ski resort. It looked like a great idea because this resort was well recognized and there was lots of potential to move around to another job if this one didn't work out.

We rented a place and settled in, and just after our first was born we bought a house and moved to the outskirts of town. Everything was amazing because he was working and I was totally focused on the family. That's all I knew and figured that's just how it was supposed to be.

Reflection - I can safely say I was happy during this time because everything was fresh and new and I was kinda just going with the flow. There are lots of things in life I need to improve on but having babies was something I seemed to be really good at.

Take Action Steps - Looking back now I see many things I would have liked to change if that was possible. Again, a lot of it would have to do with the financial. Having money would have made things easier. Now I'm not saying having money makes you happy, but it does open the door for more opportunity and certainly takes the stress out of paying your bills. I would have also worked a little harder at staying connected with my partner, instead of focusing 110 percent on being a mom. Just a few things you might want to think about if you still have the opportunity to make different choices.

Chapter Three

Marriage Breakup

"Splitting up really isn't a tragedy. The tragedy is when you decide to stay in an unhappy marriage, showing your children the wrong things about love. You aren't going to die from getting a divorce."

This factor is going to be different in every relationship. It's tough to make a marriage work and there's always going to be things you could have both done differently to perhaps change the outcome.

In some cases, marriages are essentially doomed to fail from the start. I'd like to believe nobody ever gets married to assume the marriage will eventually break.

In my case, I believed the man I was marrying was going to be with me forever. That's a dream many children have that are raised in a loving, stable family. It actually hurts the more I think because I never wanted to be the one that failed in marriage.

That's some of my family pressure creeping up on me.

Fast forward to baby number four. Up until my fourth child, it was smooth sailing for me. I took care of my body by eating right and exercising and actually seemed to get smaller with each pregnancy. Don't get me wrong, I worked at it and was rewarded by keeping my figure slim and strong. I'm sure some genetics played a part too.

Feeling good about my body helped me to feel good about being a mother and that helped me enjoy all the trials and tribulations that come with being a mom. That's my belief anyway.

So pregnancy number four was fine until my 20-week ultrasound. My heart was smashed to pieces when my doctor told me there was something wrong with the baby and it might not survive to be delivered. Worse yet, the baby might have serious defects that could take away from its quality of life.

I was broken. I needed a shoulder to lean on and positive thinking.

Unfortunately, I didn't get it. I needed answers and I was set to go to a high-risk pregnancy clinic to get them.

This was where everything started to break in my marriage. My then-husband didn't give me the understanding and hope I needed. Initially, he said, "I think we should just get rid of it." Those words are still etched in my brain.

At the time I couldn't understand. I was connected with this child and never thought for a minute about getting rid of the baby. I didn't know it at the time but I put my wall up. My belief at the time was I would never ever be able to forgive those words.

That's some of the stubborn farmer in me. I was strong and determined and willing to push forward alone if I needed to.

I kept pushing my partner away further and further and focusing more and more on the children. They were my priority.

I'm going to fast-forward again. My fourth child survived but it was many years of surgeries, medications, worries, not knowing and stress. I tried to keep it all together but realized I was so far away from my then-husband that I didn't even have the energy to try and figure things out. We were distant, more like friends for the most part.

I decided I needed to leave him only to find out I was expecting again. So much for birth control pills. They definitely didn't work for me.

I wasn't sure how I was going to tell him so I just did it. He didn't believe me and he got angry with me and rightly so I guess. That anger scared me and pushed me to stand stronger in my decision. You see all I wanted was to be loved and shown love, taken care of and cherished by that one special man.

My strong head made me believe that my kids deserved to see what my mom and dad had, and I didn't think we had it.

I struggled with the decision but at that moment in time, I felt it was the only move to make. I wasn't getting the love and support I deserved. So I wrote up the separation agreement and started the process.

At that time the kids were 8, 6, 4, and 3...around there anyway.

The only one that had a chance of understanding the breakup was my oldest boy. He was sweet and understanding and crazy smart. I told the children and I made sure they knew they were loved by both of us and no matter what mom and dad would always be friends. There was no fighting or making things difficult for each other.

We both loved the kids and for that reason we wanted our children to know this was a decision between the two of us because we want what's best for the kids.

I was crying of course and I cried harder when my 8-year-old son put his arms around me said, "Mom, don't cry. It will be okay. Maybe one day we will have two families. Wouldn't that be great!"

He said it so matter of fact that my heart ached. I was so proud of him for being so understanding and strong when I was prepared for him to get mad at me. He did the exact opposite and if it makes any sense, that made it worse.

K...I'm going to stop there or I'll be rambling on forever.

Reflection - This is one of the most difficult times in my life. Perhaps I set my standards and expectations in my marriage too high? My partner wanted simple and I wanted "more." I was following my heart which I often did. Perhaps I should have used a little more logic.

Emotions and logic just don't mix.

I did what I thought was right but maybe I should have put more thought into everything.

Take Action Steps - This is where I would suggest getting a marriage counselor or talking to a therapist. We never tried that and frankly the thought never even occurred to me. Again, that's a little bit of the farmer in me. I was brought up to believe seeing a counselor was a sign of weakness and I think you know by now I believed I was basically allergic to weakness.

I now believe every couple should talk regularly with a therapist just to help keep things on track and work through issues with guidance. I learned this lesson the hard way.

Chapter Four

Personal Internal Struggles

"If you choose to try and please everyone but yourself, you are setting yourself up for a life of endless struggles."

It's tough sometimes to admit your weaknesses. Tougher still to admit when you've made a mistake. I can safely say my personal internal struggles were all interconnected with failure. Something I was taught never to do as a child. I was so strong and worked so hard to reach my goals that I didn't "fail" very often. Yes, I certainly screwed up, but there's a ginormous difference between failing and screwing up, for me anyway.

Screwing up is making a mistake and learning from it. For instance, I screwed up when I forgot to put the cap on the milk tank and I flooded the milk house. I did that once, learned from it, and put it behind me.

Failing to me is about falling short in an expectation to someone else. I'm pretty sure I shouldn't think this way but I do.

I felt like a failure as a daughter, wife, and parent.

All of which means the world to me. Disappointing the people I love is worse for me than breaking an arm or a leg.

Failure As A Daughter

My dad was/is my hero. He taught me to be strong, not to cry and to put in the time and energy to be the best. His expectations of me were huge and I worked hard to make sure I delivered every time. He always used to say I always did the opposite of what he suggested.

I didn't do this on purpose but I can see where he's coming from.

There were no divorces in my family at the time. I felt completely broken knowing I was going to be the first to get divorced. On top of that, I know my dad is focused on making sure you've got financial stability. Of course, I didn't have that. I felt like I failed him on so many levels because of what he wanted for me, his strong daughter.

I felt weak and that too was a failure in my mind. I can't help the way I felt/feel.

I remember dating a man that was willing to take care of me and my children completely. On many levels, he was great for me. He loved to surprise me. Built me a house for me and my children. He was always one step ahead of me for the things I needed.

However, he was unbalanced and that caused a whole bunch of issues with me. I didn't want my kids seeing certain sides of him and his anger really did scare me.

I left and my father made it clear how disappointed he was in me. Yes, I was going back to nothing but at least I had myself and my children. All I wanted to do was to rebuild and eventually find the man of my dreams that "fit" with me.

To this day my father still believes I was silly to leave this man just because he was financially stable. What about my internal happiness? The stress of this helped push me to make poor decisions. To not follow my heart and my gut and realize this was MY life to live and I deserved to be happy. I didn't and don't need the approval of anyone to tell me what makes me happy.

I've learned that the difficult way. It still breaks my heart that he feels this way but there are some things I will always protect my family from knowing for all the right reasons. I made the right decision regardless of the fact I chose a heartbreakingly difficult path.

Failure As A Wife

Like I mentioned before, nobody gets married expected to get a divorce. I spent many nights awake wondering what I should have done to stay connected. Or perhaps I just married the wrong man. Of course, I wouldn't change a thing no matter how much it hurt because I wouldn't have my beautiful children if I did.

I remember feeling like the weight of the world was on my shoulders and I didn't know which way to turn.

You see, when you are brought up believing in fairy tales and happily ever afters, it's tough to imagine that it won't end that way with you. I remember dreaming as a little girl of finding my Prince Charming and happily building a life together that would last till the end of time.

That wasn't to be and at that time my heart just wasn't feeling it. I wanted to care and love more and I didn't. It was like a switch was turned off and I couldn't ignore it. This is what I wanted to feel my any means but it truly was what I felt.

I was battling myself internally as to whether I should fake it and stay put for the sake of my children or reach for the stars to find what I believed I deserved. I am a dreamer.

This didn't make it hurt any less. I hate hurting people, period. I felt I had to do it and I did. My actions and the consequences I will have to face for the rest of my life. And being stubborn doesn't help the scenario at all.

Failure As A Parent

This was the one that hurt the worst. My kids at the time were extremely supportive and understanding but I knew it wasn't that simple. Children that come from broken families, even if it's civil, have more emotional and mental challenges than children brought up in a solid home.

The best I could do was to make sure we provided as much stability as we could. Although not having their father in the house was going to affect the kids whether I wanted to admit it or not. I felt like I was putting myself before the children but for my reasons, I needed to.

I guess the kids were too young to really understand. They still saw their father, he just didn't live with us. Throughout our marriage he worked crazy hours, so it was me that was with them 90% of the time, that's just the way it was.

No blame, I thought that was just the way it was supposed to go.

It's just tough when you only know families that stick together through thick and thin. But what about those couples that stay together for the sake of the children and they really aren't happy? Is that the right thing to do?

I felt I was stronger than that and I wanted to try and show my children you only learn by doing. It's impossible to control the feeling and actions of another person. Sure, you might love them but what if they change in a negative manner? Are you still supposed to stick with them through thick and thin?

I think no matter how difficult it is, you are stronger when you decide to walk away when you don't have your whole heart in the relationship. That's just me, always taking the long route around.

Reflection - It's ok to feel. It's okay to cry. I didn't know that when I was struggling internally. I would cry at night silently when I knew I was alone. That way I could be bright and positive and strong for my children. Their complete happiness means everything to me. I didn't want people to feel bad because I was struggling.

In other words, I tried to deal with everything alone. I shut everyone out when I should have let them in to help guide me and tell me everything was going to be okay.

I wasn't Super Woman but I was trying to be her. I should have got some help with my internal struggles. That's not weak, I see that now. In fact, that would have made me even stronger.

Take Action Steps - Once again you only know what you know. Take action to talk to people about what you are struggling with inside. Don't keep it deep inside and try to handle it on your own.

Give yourself permission to "feel." If you are sad you can be sad. If you are angry you can feel angry. Acknowledge your feelings and move on with a positive focus the best you can.

There are people that love you and WANT to help you feel better. There are going to be cloudy days but that doesn't mean you don't deserve the sunshine too.

Chapter Five

Finding Balance

"Issues arise when trying to find a balance between what others need from you and what you need just for yourself."

One of the most difficult challenges I face as a single mom is allowing myself to find a balance between doing for me and for my children. For almost 18 years it was ALL about my kids. It wasn't until recently that I started giving myself permission to give to me too.

If you don't take care of you, how are you going to be able to be an amazing mom?

Trust me, I totally screwed up with this one because I know a happy mom is a good mom.

I made sure I had an hour each day to exercise, that was for me. Other than that I really did nothing. I didn't buy clothes, get my hair done or go to the spa. For me, that was the guilt card and it made me feel bad. Simply because there was always something the kids needed and in my mind, they came first.

That's true, but only too a point.

When my daughter was at Sick Kid's fighting for her life for her first three months of life, I was at the hospital meeting the surgeons at 6 in the morning every day, and I didn't leave till 7 at night. I felt I needed to be punished I guess for her struggles even though I had nothing to do with it. I felt I should have been able to protect her from all the surgeries, pocks and prodding, but I couldn't. Her life was in the hands of her doctors and medical team.

Once again I felt like a failure. I shut everyone out and tried to deal with it all on my own. I had no balance. One hour a day I allowed myself to exercise like crazy but that was it.

That's just one example of me not being balanced.

Another is never leaving the kids with a sitter to go out for the evening. I always had my kids with me, even when I went for my doctor's appointment. They would sit quietly in the waiting room until I was done. Amazing children I have but I was never able to find the balance between giving to me and to my children.

I didn't even let my mom stay with me for a few weeks after my first boy was born. She came to see him and I tried to do it all on my own. Balance would have been to let her stay with me and help me. Instead, I thought I needed to "do it all" and I know I hurt her in the process. Sorry, mom for trying to be so strong.

When you are a single mom raising children, balance is vital. Don't make the same mistakes I did because you deserve to be happy and so do your children. Find things that make you happy and lean on the people that you love to help you make them a part of your daily life.

The more balanced you are in the big picture, the better it will be for everyone.

Reflection - This is one place where I would do things differently if I could. I would force myself to give me permission to do for "mom" too. I didn't have to "do it all." I deserved to get my nails done, go out for dinner, or to get pampered at the spa on occasion. Find your balance and understand you don't have to do it all. Even if it's just going out for a coffee with a friend.

Take Action Steps - I can't stress how important it is for you to focus on balance in whatever struggles you are dealing with as a single mom. Make the time for you so that you can be stronger for your kids. Don't be stubborn like me and give yourself permission to take care of you.

It's important you understand you deserve too. Do me a favor and make a point of doing something for just you each and every day. I screwed up here and that was a large factor in what was breaking me down. Just trust me on this one, please.

Chapter Six

Back Into Dating

"When you forgive yourself you open up the door to a brand new amazing beginning."

There is no right or wrong time to get back into dating after a divorce. You just need to step out there when you are ready and give it a shot.

After my official divorce, it was about two years before I had a coffee date with another man. Yes, it was weird at first, but I enjoyed getting out of "mom mode" if you know what I mean. I started with an online "meeting." That's what I called it anyway to take the pressure off. To me, dating was when you've already met a guy and been out at least a few times, deciding to see if you can make things work.

It's really important that you step outside your comfort zone and try dating again after your separation or divorce. You deserve to be happy completely and your child or children also deserve to see that.

The last thing I wanted to do was to have my children think that "marriage" can't work. Just because it didn't work for mom doesn't mean it can't work for each of them.

I also want them to know that you only know by doing and if you wind up with someone and it's just not working out, it's okay to figure out what's best for you. You can't fail by trying. I spent most of my life believing I had to succeed in everything. That's both good and bad but it's also freaking crazy. Follow your gut and use a little logic and you will do just fine.

My issue with dating was that I wound up with too many potentials. Probably because I tend to ignore the negative and look for the positive. I never met with a really "wrong" man. I saw potential in many and with my optimistic attitude that was a recipe for disaster. Not to mention the fact I'm really shitty at making decisions.

What I will say is that there are no set proven rules as to when you should jump back into the big bad world of dating after breaking up. More importantly, make sure you don't hide away just because.

Another important lesson I learned was to wait to introduce the kids to this new man of yours. Never forget their eyes are watching you 24/7. You need to help strengthen their belief in a healthy, happy relationship. Take your time and make sure you are ready to take things to the next level before you let your children meet him. Something I learned the tough way.

If you aren't comfortable with online dating don't be afraid to let some of your trusted friends set you up. There's no harm in meeting men with common interests and taking it from there.

My thinking, you never know unless you try. Don't rush it but having another support in the mix will help you deal with all the tough and sometimes beautiful challenges you will face as a single mom. Just my thinking...

Reflection - I think I waited just about the right time before stepping back into the dating scene. It's stressful when you adding another to your plate. I learn by doing and that's exactly what I did.

Just understand you shouldn't have to try and make him fit. If your gut is telling you there are a few red flags, follow your gut. Long-term relationships are tough with perfect conditions and you deserve to be loved for you. Don't let your past relationship patterns sabotage your future relationships.

Take Action Steps - Slow and steady wins the race here. The only rules are the ones you make. You deserve what you want and you shouldn't settle for anything less. Stand strong and understand if you need to you can raise your children on your own.

Believe in your internal strength. Follow your heart and go after what you want. You will do just fine.

Chapter Seven

Getting Help - Letting In

"It's impossible to think you can help everyone, but there is someone everyone can reach out to and help."

This is another tough one for me because I was taught at a young age to do it all on my own, otherwise, I was weak. This isn't necessarily a bad thing, however, when reality hits you will get smacked.

Can you believe I didn't get any real counseling until more than 5 years after my divorce? Silly me...please don't make the same mistake because another ear can't hurt.

You are only human and you can only handle so much. Don't take it all on alone as I did.

When you are a single mom you are essentially acting as mom and dad the best you can. That's a lot of stress and it's very important you open up and get some advice on the decisions you are going to make for you and your kids.

I didn't have any reflection or help for the most part. Yes, I had a couple of friends I checked in with occasionally, but that wasn't enough, I see that now.

It's hard enough to raise kids with two parents in our world today, let alone as a single mom. This is just a fact, not good or bad. I never even thought to seek out any sort of counseling to help me with my day to day struggles. I kept it all to myself and let it build up until I was literally ready to implode.

If you've got a supportive X that's a bonus. However, if you are fighting back and forth you need to understand that is causing irreversible damage to your children. Try not to damage your kids because of the adult choices you've made. We can't reverse time so make sure you make smart choices with that.

Having a neutral counselor in your corner is a good thing because they will help you to make a better choice for you and your family. Something to think about.

Reflection - One of my worst missteps was not getting professional help or guidance when I should have. I was built with a super tough skin. That's not something I should be proud of. The strongest people are the ones that accept and look for help. That's the truth.

Take Action Steps - If I could take different steps I would look to getting some help with my decisions. I need to tell you it's okay to get some help. You are perfectly fine to talk with someone about what's bothering you. I was taught to be closed. Please be open. It's only going to help you find yourself and get stronger.

Chapter Eight

Time For Me

I'm not sure this fits in but I will say it's really important as a single mom that you find time for just you. That means no kids, nothing else. I understand this is a tough pill to swallow. Start small and go from there.

It might just be 20 minutes for a coffee alone down the street to start, that's okay. If you love to read you can find a quiet spot to get lost in a book. It really doesn't matter what you do just as long as you do things for yourself on a daily basis.

I made the mistake of making pretty much no time for me and I paid for that. You can give to your children but you still deserve. Please just trust me on that and promise me you won't feel guilty. I've been a mom for 20 years now and I'm still working on this.

Being a single mom is the toughest job in the world but you WILL be a better mom if you make time for you. It doesn't have to be much but you do need to do something for you.

One issue I still battle with is finding excuses not to put the focus on me. The bills are always going to be there. The cleaning will never end. And of course, your children are probably pressing you for every second they can. That's ok, just set your limitations.

Let your kids know beforehand when you are going to not be available for them and why. Be straight up and tell them you need a little time just for you because you want to be the best mom ever. If you can have a babysitter or a friend or family member commit to taking over for you on a scheduled basis, that's perfect.

Give yourself something to look forward to. I find that helps me to get through some of the difficult challenges that seem to find me.

The only rule I have for you is no kids allowed.

Reflection - Tough as always was how I was brought up. That's not necessarily right. I know I should have made time for me, for mom, to find a little more balance. If I could reverse time I would have let my mom watch the kids for a day or two. I would have let a babysitter look after the kids so I could go out and interact with adults. I never did, my bad.

Take Action Steps - My advice here would be for you as a single mom, to make sure you take time for just you. That means you need to accept help from your family and friends to help with your kids.

You deserve what you want. You deserve to be happy. That's all I've got to say here.

Chapter Nine

Overcoming Guilt

"As humans, we tend to focus on negative things more than the positive. Inevitably your mind gets obsessed with negative things, judging, guilt and anxieties, that are created from your thoughts about the future and so much more."

Straight up...guilt consumes me. That's the truth. I always wanted my children to grow up in a concrete, stable environment. I failed in that and for that, I am truly sorry. I have amazing kids but I will always carry the guilt because I didn't make it easier.

My children don't have a "mom and dad" together and I will live with that forever.

The guilt really can't be overcome but I want you to know, nobody should judge anyone else. We all have our screw-ups. We've all made mistakes. My belief is that nobody can judge anyone else unless they agree to walk in their shoes.

Guilt is something that comes with every single mom on the planet. Accept that and try to not let it take over. You are only one person and you can only do what you can do. There's a lot to be said for you working 24/7 to make sure everyone is okay.

For years I felt guilty, I still do. The fact is that really doesn't help things, the guilt is not productive for me.

What you really need to do after experiencing it all, is to just try and do the best you can and not feel guilty at all for it.

It seems really quite simple.

I understand families come in all different shapes and sizes and as long as there is love and support, all "families" can be happy and healthy. That doesn't mean it still didn't hurt when one of my children would come home and talk about one of their friends and what they were going to be doing on the weekend with their mom and dad.

I tried hard not to let that derail me but it was just one of those things I never got used to. Got me wondering "what if," sometimes.

Reflection - Guilt is something that will eat you from the inside out. Please don't let it. Mind over matter here. You need to stand strong because I know you are strong. Guilt will always be there...I know that...I live it.

Take Action Steps - Everyone faces guilt, particularly single moms in my opinion. Family is important and when it's been broken you can't help but feel responsible. I want you to keep your guilt feelings in perspective and try to channel them positively.

It's time to put the past behind you, release your guilt and let it go. It's not going to be easy but you can do it, I know you can.

Chapter Ten

Dealing With Unbalanced Family Dynamics

"Life is just like riding a bike. You've got to keep your balance and keep on peddling."

When you lose your balance you're going to fall. I don't think you can have balance in the family dynamics when you are a single mom. You can't be mom and dad. You can try like I did but you'll still be unbalanced.

For me, it was tough dealing with the scheduling of when the kids would see their father and what new role he would play in their lives. Although I was with the kids pretty much 24/7 in their younger years, I understood and believed in the importance of having their father in their lives as much as possible.

The only reason I wouldn't let that happen was if I felt the kids weren't safe with him or he was into some serious legal troubles. Thankfully, none of which applied for me.

It was very important my children saw that their dad loved them. And the only way to really show that to a child beyond the shadow of a doubt is to spend time with them. Buying them gifts or sending them off on trips without you, just isn't going to cut it down the road.

You might be very angry with your ex but it's important the children don't see this or feel it. Sure, there will be times when you say or do things you shouldn't try and hurt your ex. Just make sure it's an exception to the rule. If you are constantly battling with your ex you are knowingly causing irreversible damage to your children and they don't deserve that.

We had to work on planning separate Christmases. I was pretty lucky I guess because my ex wasn't into the holidays too much and usually just made an appearance at some point. We never had to seek legal counsel to help figure out the family dynamics. Good thing because we didn't have the money to do that.

In some cases, you might need to get legal advice to figure out what's fair for everyone. To me, that's very sad but true. I've heard of some pretty nasty divorces that put the kids and the rest of the family through hell.

Do what you need to do to find a new balance in your life, it's important.

Reflection - It seems like I'm always struggling to find balance in my life. I knew how important it was, particularly when my divorce was fresh, that we tried to maintain a balance in our family. Things were changing fast but reassuring our children everything would be okay and establishing at least an outline of a family platform really did help.

Take Action Steps - Work with your ex to find a new balance. Neither of you has to like it but you need to deal with it for the sake of the kids. You don't want them to be the victims here for your choices. They deserve to smile and so do you. Which makes it that much more important that you take action to keep things as close as you can to normal for your kids. You can. You will.

Chapter Eleven

No Blame

"You are better to accept responsibility rather than assigning blame. Allow the possibilities to inspire you and lift you up, not beat you up and discourage."

This is a tough chapter to write. Nobody goes into a relationship thinking it's going to end; that's just not how it works. What's tough to let go of is the blame, for me anyway. It's so easy to point the finger, to feel like all of your family issues rest on your shoulders.

It will take time, but you the parent, must not take the blame for everything. In time your children will try and make you feel guilty about things that happened years ago, most of which you aren't even conscious of.

What you need to remember is that blaming is easy. Looking for solutions and accepting responsibility for your actions, within reason, is not. This means your children too need to step up to the plate and deal with the internal issues they have brewing inside of them.

Initially, I blamed myself when my marriage broke up, regardless of the fact it takes two to tango. Years went by and I learned to deal with it. Then suddenly my children were older and a few of them, two in my case, my oldest daughters, started to act out and point the finger at me for everything.

Broke my heart but no matter what I did, I finally realized I would be blamed. They were looking for a scapegoat and I was it. I was the trigger for their anger and frustrations. All of their internal issues of conflict that were never dealt with were going to be blamed on me if I gave them the opportunity.

A mother's natural instinct is to try and fix things, which doesn't work if you have a marriage breakdown and your children haven't really learned how to accept the facts and move on. By trying to talk with them, text them, or have any sort of relationship with them, I was playing into their game of hurt and allowing them to use me as the guilty punching bag.

By trying to help them I was engaging and pushing their trigger button. The that unfortunately came across and hurtful, hateful rage.

What you need to remind yourself is that all children deal with a marriage breakup differently. You might think that you've explained everything to them and that it's all okay. But that might not be the case.

It could very well be years before your children have the ability to face their fears and internal hurts. And if they choose not to deal with them, you might very well be the one that gets to pay the ultimate price, a serious disconnect with your children.

Sad and heartbreaking but totally true.

If you've only got one child then you might not have such a huge challenge. Having the ability to focus on just one child is normally easier than focusing on many. In my case, I have six. Each at different stages of intellect and each with very different methods of dealing with their feelings.

Some of them just bottle the feelings up deep inside and they just sit and simmer until they are ready to explode, instead of talking them through early on. My boys seem to have a better grasp on their emotions and they learned how to ask the questions they needed to ask and come to terms with their feelings towards both me and their father.

I'm lucky they are generally supportive toward both of us.

I'm also lucky I am still on the same page with my ex. We don't trash talk to each other and we essentially support each other's actions as much as we can.

I know I'm rambling a little bit. I just want to make sure you understand that guilt card or blame card can only go so far. It's not fair for you to take the blame forever. It's all about stepping up to the plate and dealing with the circumstance, finding and being given forgiveness, and moving on.

Reflection - This was likely and still is the most difficult issue for me being a single mother. You want your children to never hurt and of course, you don't want to hurt either. Well, you don't really have control over this one.

*You only control you, nobody else.

This means if your child is going to choose to not deal with their internal questions at the time of your breakup, there's not a lot you can do about it. Especially if you don't find out about it until years down the road.

If I could do this one differently I would, starting with counseling immediately, even if you think everything is okay.

Take Action Steps - My strong advice to you would be to find some local support services to help your children and yourself, your family unit, work through your marriage breakup issues. Children don't want their mom and dad to separate. They want mom and dad to stay together forever.

Unfortunately, this isn't the case too much of the time.

Even if you think counseling isn't needed, do it anyway.

Why?

It's going to make sure you avoid harsh realities that might arise down the road. Hurtful feelings that have been buried under the carpet that will eventually surface with a vengeance. Prevention is everything here.

Chapter Twelve

Accepting Professional Help

"When you accept help from someone it doesn't mean you're a failure. All it means is you just aren't alone."

A huge mistake I made was not accepting the professional help I needed, and my children, until too much damage was done.

As a single mother, you can't possibly know everything. You can't expect yourself to naturally know how to fix the hurt triggered by a marriage breakup. It really doesn't matter the circumstances. It's tough to look outside the box from all angles when you are cornered inside.

You are trying to do everything you can to make sure your children don't hurt, but you can't do this alone. You need to enlist the help of professional counselors.

Believe me, I tried big time to do this alone and I'm afraid I failed miserably.

Tap into the social services in your community and get the counseling you need. Make sure there are professionals your children can reach out to that are going to be there to guide them through the process of dealing with their family breakup.

This is something you can't do alone. I know I said this before but I'm saying it again.

 grew up programmed to take care of everyone and everything. This meant I never really reached out to anyone else for advice, other than my friends I guess and that was no a casual basis.

We live in a very complex world with a crazy amount of stress. It's not like you live off the land and only have to worry about good weather for the crops. The technology and lack of human interaction are in large part a cause for our excess stressful world.

Talking with someone outside of your social circle is only going to help. Getting the professional opinion of a trained counselor can help you to take steps in the right direction and feel better about yourself and your situation.

Open your mind to this. There are lots of free social programs within your community that will show you how to get some help. At least a person to bounce your thoughts off of. Give it a shot.

Reflection - As I've already mentioned, this is where I royally screwed up. I wanted to try and do it all and that caused more damage than not. I thought I had eventing under control but I didn't know enough to ask the right questions to all of my children. Some of them seemed to get it and others not so much.

This is too important to ignore.

Take Action Steps - This one is pretty self-explanatory. Take action to tap into as many professional counseling services as you can. You can never get too much help when it comes to undoing the damage that has already been done when any mom and dad break up, particularly when your children are too young to really know what's going on.

Chapter Thirteen

Difficult Emotional Challenges And Solutions

"Something I learned the hard way was that it doesn't help to get down on yourself. Make sure you keep and take action by making optimism a way of life so you can believe in yourself again." CAW

It's safe to say being a single mom comes with numerous difficult emotional challenges that present themselves and prove to be overwhelming. From feeling guilt and lack of confidence to money and the stress of making decisions solo, there is hope, there are solutions.

Emotions and logic don't physiologically mix. In other words, they can't occur simultaneously. For me, that means if I'm emotionally charged, I'm not going to make the best logical decisions. What I want you to understand is that you are not alone. Every other mom out there facing these numerous emotional challenges to different degrees.

Here are a few that come to mind because I've experienced them and have tried to keep them under control.

Challenge One - Doubting Yourself

It's very difficult to know if you are doing a good job as a mom when you don't have someone beside you to remind you. I know it doesn't take long for my mind to start doubting my ability as a single mom. And when the doubt creeps in my insecurities skyrocket.

Sure, my friends and sometimes my family would remind me that I was doing a good job, but for me, that's not as effective as having a partner to reassure me I was on the right track.

On the flip side of that having a partner tell you when you've fallen short or just pointing out better ways to handle things, is a huge plus.

You are not alone if you start feeling self-doubt.

Solution

Something that helped me was to get out of the house and get involved with other young moms. Joining some sort of walk-in club with moms and kids is a great way to start feeling more secure in your parenting skills.

I became inspired by other moms and learned lots. Tell yourself every day that nobody is perfect and that you've got to be doing something right because you've got happy kids.

Try taking a deep breath, have a good cry if you need to, and remind yourself you are doing the best job you can.

Challenge Two - Hurting When The Kids Are With Their Father

I was with my children 24/7, so it was extremely difficult when the kids went with their father. The loneliness that set in took a lot out of me and I don't think I ever really got used to it. As much as they could drive me crazy and I told myself I needed a break, the minute they were gone I wanted them back.

In my situation, they never really went for more than a day, but that doesn't make this emotional challenge any easier. The first time they went with their dad I remember busying myself cooking and cleaning and getting ready for them to come back.

Looking back now I see that I should have used that time for me and filled it with things I wanted to do. I should have read a good book and grabbed a good nap, but I didn't.

Solution

One of the easiest strategies to stay clear of the missing is to get busy. This is the time to schedule a coffee date with a friend or maybe go out to dinner and to a club. Do the things you can't really do when you have your children with you.

This way you will have a little fun without missing your kids too much. You deserve the break and spending time on you.

Challenge Three - Money Stress

I would stay this is the one factor the could time and again completely suck the life out of me. I tried to keep the money worries to myself but it's tough when that was my reality. I had times where I could only put three dollars of gas in my car and hope we made it to our destination.

What really hurt me was there were so many things I wanted my children to have, that they deserved to have, and they had to do without because I just didn't have the money. I always seemed to be behind in the bills and there was always more going out than there was coming it.

I felt my ex should have supported us more because I was the one raising the children. That really didn't happen and I tried to pick up the slack with writing. Burning the candle at both ends just doesn't work. All it does is burn you out and stress you more.

Solution

Where there's a will there's a way.

Truth be told, as long as there is food on the table and a roof over your head, you are doing okay. That's what I told myself. I also made sure I got a workout in at least 5 days a week. Often it was just at home but when I exercise my mind settles and I just don't worry so much.

Try creating a budget and looking for ways to cut your spending. Just be sure you don't become too frugal or you will feel deprived. I used to put any change in my pockets into a jar on top of the fridge. I used that as extra found money. When it hit a certain point I would take the kids out for an ice-cream or maybe even for dinner.

I think that was more for my brain but knowing there was some change on top of the fridge no matter how money stressed I felt, was peace of mind for me.

Challenge Four - There's Nobody To Take Over

I can't tell you how many days I was just exhausted or wasn't feeling well and the only choice I had was to pick myself up and keep on going. When you don't have a partner you can't have any timeouts. There's nobody there to pass the parenting duties onto when you just need a little nap after being up half the night with the baby.

When I was feeling like this was also when I started doubting myself about leaving in the first place. Honestly, there were times where I thought I should have just stuck it out in my relationship only so I could get a little break now and again. I know that wasn't logical but that's how I felt.

Stay strong, I know you are.

Solution

Take a deep breath, close your eyes, and remind yourself you can do it and you just need a minute to calm yourself and gather your thoughts. If you really need a minute just put on a video for the kids to watch or put them to sleep.

It's much better to do that instead of letting yourself get angry at them.

This was a little sneaky but sometimes I would just move the clock ahead a couple of hours and put the kids to bed so I could have some alone time. A little more sleep never hurts them that's for sure.

Challenge Five - Making Every Decision On Your Own

For me, making decisions is seriously tiring. Some days all I wanted was for someone else to make all the decisions. I really didn't care what they were I just didn't want to make any of them.

Decision making is stressful because if you make the wrong decision, it's all on you. It didn't matter whether it was figuring out which sport to sign them up for or what kind of phone plan I should sign up for, being the only one to make the final decision was a very difficult pill for me to swallow.

Even when I got advice from family or friends I knew it was me that got the final say.

Solution

Try telling yourself that no matter what you decide, in the end, it will all work out. When you force yourself to trust your intuition and believe you are going to make a good decision, that helps to take the stress out of the decision-making process.

Look at this as a positive thing where there's no negotiating. What you say is how it's going to be and you can use this to empower yourself. You are the one in charge. You are the one in control.

This is another instance where it's mind over matter. Trust yourself and tell yourself you CAN do it.

Challenge Six - Accepting Things Didn't Go As Planned

As you know, I was raised in a healthy two-parent household. More than anything that's what I always wanted for my children.

It wasn't to be.

For a long time, I had nightmares about this. Feeling like I totally failed my children as a mom and not knowing how I was going to make things right. This is something I knew I needed to get out of my brain because as long as my kids knew they were loved, as long as I was doing my best, that was the right thing for my family.

I was worried the kids might resent me because their dad wasn't around. Lucky for me that wasn't the case. I didn't want to fill my kids in on the details specifically of why I wasn't with their father because I didn't want to burden them further. In my brain, that is adult stuff and it doesn't need to be put into the mind of a child to stress them further.

Solution

It is what it is.

What I did here was mentally prepare myself for the questions that I believed my children would one day ask me about their dad. What you need to understand is there is no absolute definition of a family. They come in all shapes and sizes.

A family is what you make it be. It can consist of friends, brothers, sisters, and partners.

When you open your mind and your arms to what you have as a family, this emotional worry will become controllable.

Challenge Seven - Losing Yourself

There's no doubt, I always felt like I had to be superwoman because there was nobody else in the picture really to help. With so much on your plate, it's super easy to forget about taking care of yourself at all.

Life is all about give and take and everyone deserves, especially single moms.

You work hard and deserve a little bit of pampering. Sometimes you've got to get clever about it but you can make the time to take care of you. It's important that you do so you can take care of your family.

I remember a time where I didn't have any extra money and I decided I needed to pamper myself with a mud mask after the kids were in bed. Guess what I did? I actually went outside, scooped up some mud from a mud puddle and proceeded to treat myself to a wrinkle-reducing mud mask.

As silly as that sounds it made me feel better.

Then I had a nice hot bath and slipped into bed.

That's all I needed to recharge just enough to get ready for the next obstacle.

Solution

It's important to take at least an hour out of the week to do something special for yourself. Go for a drive, a walk, or writing in your journal. Anything that is going to help take your mind off of your daily grind.

You need to make an effort to reconnect with you.

Challenge Eight - Extreme Fatigue

Fact...You are doing alone what is clearly a two-person job. You aren't just imagining that you are feeling physically, emotionally and spiritually pooched. What you need to understand is that your kids need you and this means you have to recognize your limitations. You need to work on understanding when you've had enough and focus on stepping back for a few minutes and taking care of you.

Solution

Get creative and think of ways to take a deep breath. I remember a few times where I dipped into the extra change on top of the fridge and hired the girl across the street for a couple of hours to watch the kids while I went for a run. That was one way I could destress and calm my brain.

Other times I would put the kids in their rooms with a few toys and I'd grab a power nap. It really doesn't matter what you do. Just make sure you address yourself before you become extremely fatigued. Do it for the sake of your children.

Chapter Fourteen

Pointers To Flip Your Switch Positive

"I will stay calm when the moment is stressful. I will let positivity escape from me in thought and action to create amazing."

It's not hard to fall prey to negative thinking. When you allow your negative thoughts to unfold that will only bring you sadness. Everyone experiences this at some point in their life.

Your negative thinking will steal your energy and block you from being "there" in the moment. Negative energy feeds off of negative thinking. The more you allow your negative thoughts to creep into the picture, the more strength they gain.

I think of this as a snowball rolling down the hill. The further it rolls the bigger it gets.

I consider myself to be a positive thinker in general. I'm usually pretty good at pushing negative thoughts out of my brain. Although it was certainly more challenging for me after I took on the role of a single mom.

I remember laying awake many nights worrying about just about everything. Sometimes the negatives would overwhelm me and leave me feeling hopeless. I guess that's a natural part of life. I know it takes a strong person to recognize negativity and push it away.

It's very important you learn how to take control and get rid of your negative thoughts because they become destructive.

Having just one negative thought can easily turn into a negative experience before you know it. I remember one time when I was in school and my parents were coming down to visit me. I really didn't want them too because I was supposed to go away with friends. I was thinking about how bored I was going to be and I allowed my brain to keep telling me I was going to have a crappy time.

I let my negative thoughts take control.

Needless to say, my parents arrived and I was a total grump. Of course, they had no idea why I was being difficult, which of course didn't sit well with them. What could have been a really fun weekend wound up getting cut short. They left a day early and that made us both feel worse.

I ruined the weekend with one negative thought.

Here are a few pointers to help you avoid negative thinking as a single mom and push positive thoughts to the center of the stage.

Pointer One - Simply Smile

This is a tough one when you are feeling totally stressed out and tired. I have had to literally put myself in front of the mirror and force myself to smile at times. It seems a little ridiculous but it works.

Flashing those pearly whites truly does help you kick the negative thinking out the door. I also know that you use less muscles to smile than you do to frown.

Pointer Two - Reach Out And Lift Someone Up

When you take the focus off of yourself and your situation and you take positive action to help someone else, you're going to feel good. Even though I always seemed to have my plate overloaded, I could take the time to do something to help another person out when I was feeling bummed myself.

Often I would take the kids into the nursing home to visit with the elderly. I loved it when I saw their eyes light up when my children started asking them matter-of-fact questions.

Pointer Three - Take Responsibility For You

When I'm feeling really sad or unhappy I try and remind myself there is someone out there that has it tougher than me. Try not to play the victim and take responsibility for your decisions.

You only control you, nobody else.

There is always another path to take, a door to open, and there is always another way out. You will always have the choice to change things. Try and see that as a positive thinking move.

Pointer Four - Just Dance

I'm not sure where I read this but I know that people who listen to music and/or dance, are happier in general. That's my understanding anyway.

When I need to pick my mood up I love to crank up the music and do some silly singing and dancing. And believe me, you don't have to be good at either. I'm an okay dancer but my singing is awful.

Point is, I have fun with it and always feel better after. Especially when my kids are laughing at me and singing and dancing too. Singing is emotionally healing and dancing helps release your positive energy endorphins that physiologically flip your mood positive.

Pointer Five - Meditation

Meditating is a great way to stop thinking and bring your attention to focus just on your breathing. It will slow your heart rate and calm your brain. Even if you just practice some deep breathing you will be able to push your destructive thoughts away and make room for good thoughts.

This works for me when I'm feeling anxious, upset, scared, or any other extreme emotion. The great thing is you can do it anywhere and it only takes a couple of minutes.

Pointer Six - Yoga

Yoga works along the lines of meditation, with a physical component to it. This calming exercise is totally relaxing and that helps to ease the negativity in your head. Yoga keeps you in the now so you stop fretting about what "could" happen.

Back in the day, I had yoga videos I would do. Sometimes I just had time to do 10 or 15 minutes of a class, but that always helped. Today you can just watch them on U-tube or your computer if you like.

Even better would be to sign up for yoga classes and use this excuse for some "me" time to help keep you out of the negative zone.

Pointer Seven - Hang Out With Positive People

Negative breeds the negative. I have this weird thing I do when I go into a coffee shop to do some writing. If I feel a person is negative that's sitting near me, I always get up and move to another table. It may just be in my head but I know that if you hang around negativity, you will become more negative yourself.

A person's negative energy will try and steal your positive energy.

If you are thinking negative thoughts call up a friend who you know will be supportive and positive. When you are feeling down and you engage with positive people, this will help to put a smile on your face or at least a positive spin on whatever you happen to be dealing with.

Pointer Eight - Lighten Up Your Negative Tone

This is something you've got to learn to do consciously. When you are thinking about something in a negative fashion. Try and make your thought more positive. This doesn't mean the negative issue is going to be cured, but it will help you take the stress off and perhaps provide a little hope.

For instance, instead of thinking, "How am I ever going to pay all the bills on my own," think, "I'm going to face some challenges but I know it will all work out."

It takes time to master this one but when you do, there will be a lot of negative thinking that doesn't stand a chance of manifesting into more than it really is.

Humans, in general, tend to gravitate towards the negative for some reason. Take control and stop this from happening in your life as a strong, independent single mom.

Pointer Nine - List Ten Things You Are Grateful For In This Moment

When you are grateful for things that you have right now, this helps you appreciate and think positive thoughts. My list is: my children, my health, a new book I've written, my friends, taking my kids skating, snowboarding, paying my phone bill on time, starting a new job as a nanny so I can still be with my children, my children heading off to university, and my boyfriend.

Write down your list whenever you start to feel the negative thoughts sneaking up on you. Focusing positive is only going to help you push through the tough stuff to the amazing that IS to be.

Pointer Ten - Make Habit Of Reading Positive Quotes

This is such a powerful tool. For years I have started my day out posting positive thinking quotes. I've programmed this into me and it's now habit because I get feedback from the people that read my quotes and thank me for posting them.

My thinking...There's always going to be negative crap in life. Focus on the positive stuff and the negative challenges you're facing won't seem so big.

I write quotes and put them in my calendar, on my fridge, in my purse, and even on the mirror just to make sure I don't miss them.

Chapter Fifteen

Lessons Learned From A Struggling Single Mother

"Your struggles and hardships today occur so you can win tomorrow—Never give up."

It's Christmas time and everyone seems to be emptying their bank accounts to load the tree up with the latest and greatest and most expensive gadgets for their kids. A fun time of the year getting your children excited to visit Santa, making gingerbread houses and unwrapping gifts, but unfortunately for a lot of single moms, this isn't the case.

This festive season is stressful. For me, it added to the pressure and guilt of not being able to "wow" my children with everything they wanted and deserved; at least in my mind.

I remember one year selling my car so that I could afford to give my kids a good Christmas. Silly in hindsight but making sure they were smiling on Christmas morning meant the world to me.

Your children are going to love and appreciate you for doing your best to raise them. They will learn some important life lessons that only a single mom can teach. You should be proud of yourself.

Lesson One - Don't Think...Ask For Help

I know I've touched on this already but I don't want you to make the same mistake I've made over and over. I was built so strong that asking for help, in my brain, was a sign of weakness. Now I see that asking for help is a signal of strength. If you want to learn how to do your job better you've got to ask for help. That will provide you with the opportunity to learn from other people and grow as a person.

People want to help each other. Make a point of asking for help when you need it. All that's going to do is make it easier for you.

Lesson Two - Show Me Your Grit

When you grow up in a single-parent home that didn't have a load of money, that teaches you a lot about having grit, which is an external toughness to make a better future for yourself. You don't have to be given everything on a silver platter to be successful in life, to find happiness.

I know my toughness to just figure things out no matter how difficult, has helped my kids become mentally stronger. Regardless of the fact I always felt they deserved more, they appreciated what I did for them.

I love the fact I've built extremely "tough" kids. They will make better choices than me in life and they will be amazing.

Lesson Three - Use Your Resources

You kids are going to know you are the Queen of being resourceful. If your children didn't have something, you would figure out a way to get it. Everything always had a purpose. You knew how to fix the dishwasher and figure out the electronic gadgets.

This trait will help your kids get creative and figure out how to handle all sorts of different issues in their lives.

Lesson Four - Life Definitely Isn't Easy

There's no doubt that life isn't easy. Regardless of the fact you've got lots of money or nothing, everyone faces tough daily challenges. What matters is how you face these hardships. You've taught your children to face them with their glass half full.

Lesson Five - Never Worry About What Other People Think

Truth—People are always going to judge you, I don't care who you are. People will judge you for wearing the same clothes all the time or getting food from the local food bank. People are going to judge you when you head off to school and they find out your parents aren't paying for everything.

You kids will know they will never place everyone and what's important is you do what you believe is best for your family. You don't control what other people think so it's really not worth your time to worry about it.

You've taught your kids to let the haters continue to hate while they will push forward and be great.

Lesson Five - Waste Not, Want Not

Struggling in life for me was reality. I didn't waste very much and my children have learned from that. This brings me to thoughts of my grandmother. Holy crap, she didn't waste one bite of anything.

I remember looking through her freezer where I found one bite of birthday cake frozen and 1/4 of a piece of chicken. She grew up in tough times and that taught this sweet lady to never throw anything out.

I used to use the jam jars as cups and the margarine containers for cereal bowls. Although I wasn't as extreme as my grandmother.

Be happy in the fact that you've taught your children to appreciate what they have and to waste nothing if they can help it.

Lesson Six - Never Be Afraid To Cry

As I've already mentioned, crying was something I was programmed not to do. I understood it was a sign of weakness, whereas it's the exact opposite. Nobody wants to watch their mother cry.

I always cried by myself in my bed. A few times my kids caught me but not very often.

You've taught your children that it's perfectly okay to cry things out when they need to. Letting their emotions out is a good thing.

Lesson Seven - Just Chill On The Porch

This is something you see more often than not in the poorer communities. This isn't to just pass the time away. Rather it's to make the time for each other to enjoy each other's company.

As a struggle single mother, you've shown your children how to appreciate the simplistic things. Just sitting not he porch and hanging out together is invaluable in the big picture of life.

Lesson Eight - Practice Being Humble

Your children have learned from you, as a single mom, that they are so far from being the little girl or boy that worried about whether or not they would get a nice dinner. Your kids will understand that anything can be taken away in a snap.

When you are jumble you appreciate exactly what you have and you won't take it for granted.

An amazing life lesson you've taught them.

Lesson Nine - Never Stop Dreaming

I know I did the best I could. And I know I was a really great mom considering the circumstances. I have always dreamed of my children and no matter how crazy my dreams seemed to be, I made sure their minds were open to going after whatever they wanted to in life.

As a single mom, you have to show your children how to dream and more importantly, never give up.

For me dreaming is everything because it opens the door of opportunity that you would never know existed if you didn't walk through it.

You are an amazing single mom for showing your children that dreaming is real and it will lead to amazing opportunities...believe it.

Lesson Ten - Never Ever Quit

When you are a single mom trying to make the best of things there are times where you are likely going to quit. Understand that's okay. When you just couldn't tackle something anymore that pushed your kids to be stronger, to try harder.

You've taught your kids if you work harder you will get more and you will never have to struggle as much as you have.

So many people lose faith and quit and that's just not an option.

You, as a single mom has taught your children this.

Lesson Eleven - Gain Freedom With Education

I'm not sure this one really works for me because I'm overly educated. However, many single moms are struggling more because of a lack of education. I have a few girlfriends that are single moms and they dropped out of high school to work at the corner store.

If your kids happen to watch you struggle through this that's not a bad thing. You are showing them courage and perseverance. Two traits that are very important in a healthy life big picture.

You may want to pursue furthering education at some point. Maybe focusing on a new career is exactly what you need to help you gain the strength you need to be the best single mom ever. Something to think about...

Chapter Sixteen

Co-Parenting Challenges

"The definition of insanity is doing the same thing and expecting different results."

It makes sense that after a divorce you want to simply cut all ties and move on with your life. That's just not how it works when you've got children together. If your kids are young you still have a lifelong connection with your ex despite how you feel about them.

You'll be left with two path choices: You can continue to be mean to each other which creates a stressful scenario for you, your ex, and your children; or you can both figure out to set your differences aside for the sake of your children and try working together.

Experts agree when you make the decision to work together parenting, your kids will have a more stable feeling with both parents, which lowers the feelings of abandonment, decreases behavioral issues, and lowers the risk for substance abuse and so much more.

When you show your children you can work together you are giving them positive role models to help strengthen their problem-solving skills.

Truth...Divorcees often harbor deep feelings of resentment due to many years of a rocky relationship.

I was lucky in the sense I had a fairly cooperative ex and we really did want what was best for the kids when all was said and done. Of course, we had our moments, we're only human, but they were few and far in between.

Make a point of sharing the decision that the welfare of your children is the most important thing in your life, so you can both start figuring out how you are going to co-parent successfully on a respectful platform.

Both of you are going to have to be on board to make it work.

Here are a few pointers to help you make your co-parenting work:

Pointer One - Choose To Keep It Professional

Two people don't even have to like each other to get along. I'm sure you've had a co-worker at some point in your life that you really didn't like and had to figure out a way to set your differences aside and get the job done.

The same thing applies here.

Especially at the beginning of our divorce, I found it to be really tough mentally to even be in the same house as my ex. My strategy was to keep if very factual and to try and keep my emotions out of it.

I guess you could say I treated it like a business. Short and sweet and to the point just enough to make sure we were on the same page as parents.

Pointer Two - Keep The Lines Of Communication Wide Open

If you want to make co-parenting work, you are going to have to communicate openly with every aspect of your children. I found face-to-face and telephone conversations the most difficult. The good news is emailing and texting is pretty much the norm these days.

I remember getting really frustrated because my ex was always calling me and I just wanted to use emailing unless it was an emergency, and then texting was allowed. Drove me freakin nuts some days.

The good news about emailing and texting is you can take an extra minute or two to read it over before you send it. Remember, the shorter the better and if you found you were getting a little heated, give yourself permission to take a breather and send it later.

It doesn't help anybody, particularly your kids if you are getting snappy with your ex.

Pointer Three - Keep Updated With The Important Things

It doesn't serve a positive purpose if you are trying to hide things from your ex about your children. If you've both got joint custody, the law says you need to make sure your ex knows what's going on when it comes to school, medical issues, etc.

I remember going through a time where I wasn't keeping my ex in the loop as much as I should have just because. It wasn't the right thing to do but I guess I just felt I was entitled to do this. Maybe I just wanted to have control and leave him wondering?

Bad move on my part.

There was no harm in shooting him an email telling him when the Christmas concert was and how they were doing in school.

Even if you don't like each other, little gestures like that are going to help give you both a certain degree of trust. Life is all about give and take. Make a point of trying to give when you can and hopefully he'll do the same in return.

Do it for the sake of your children.

Pointer Four - You've Got To Be Flexible

Even when you've got a court-ordered visitation schedule and parenting plan, there are going to be hiccups along the road. In order to keep the peace, it's vital that you keep an open mind and be flexible.

Understand there are going to be times where you aren't going to be able to take the kids and you're going to need your ex to step in. Leave the fussiness out of this and do your best to make sure you try to pick up the slack when your ex gets in a pinch.

My ex and I were pretty good with this one. If he couldn't take the kids I tried not to make a big deal about it.

The last thing you need to do is make a mountain out of a molehill. Be flexible and you will avoid building animosity between the two of you.

Pointer Five - Set Up Shared Calendars

Thank goodness for technology in this instance. Having online calendars is an excellent route to make sure you both know what's going on. Make sure you've got everything from visitations and school breaks, to medical appointments and special events.

Being organized will help you steer clear of miscommunication that's only going to lead to more stress and tension.

Off the hop, my ex and I didn't have a calendar and we did have a few issues with miscommunication. One of them that I remember clearly was when my ex was supposed to pick the kids up from indoor soccer training. They should have been home by 7 and when 7:30 rolled around I was getting worried.

I called my ex and he totally forgot. The kids were still at the gym, sitting there waiting with their coach. Boy was I peeved.

All things aside, we got ourselves set up with an online calendar and that helped us avoid miscommunication slip-ups.

Pointer Six - Try To Muster Up Ground Rules That Are Close

This is in the best interest of your children. If you both have opposite expectations and rules, your kids are going to get confused and trust me, you'll have many more battles on your hands.

You may have different parenting styles, and that's okay. But it's important that you have similar basic rules; like bedtimes and watching tv; so your kids know what is expected of them.

Make sure neither of you is the "Disney World parent" that gives you children everything and lets them do whatever they want just so you'll get their attention. That's a guilt card in most instances and it won't help your children develop in a healthy manner.

This was another pointer that used to get me ticked. Since the kids didn't see their father that often, he would randomly swoop in and take them out for ice-cream, to the park, or for some other treat. They were always so excited to see him because it was all fun and games. I was the parent at home enforcing the rules, telling them to go to bed and disciplining them.

I felt that was totally not fair.

Make sure you both figure out what the basic rules are going to be. It's going to help you show your kids you are on the same page in parenting and save you a lot of headaches.

Pointer Seven - When You Co-Parent, Conflict Needs To Vamoose

You're only human and you're not going to agree with each other 24/7. That's fine, just make sure you remember that you are working together as a team for the sake of the kids. Take action to make sure you don't have an all-out war in front of the kids because you are only hurting your kids and each other.

You are going to be challenged with this one for sure. Just remember, you are doing this for your children. Think of the stress they are under with your divorce or separation. They deserve you both to show them a loving front that is going to be supportive and understanding.

Learn to cooperate and use your manners and your children will benefit from it.

I guess I was lucky in the fact that my ex really didn't like any sort of confrontation. Very rarely did he lose it.

We all know it takes two to tango.

I'm not going to lie, there were a few times where we pushed each other's buttons and said things we shouldn't have. For that I'm sorry. The good news is he would usually let me vent and not come back at me. Which meant the conversation was over, no harm done.

Chapter Seventeen

The Do's And The Don'ts About Talking To Kids About Divorce

"Divorce means there are going to be changes. I used to think of divorce as a failure but now I see it as an opportunity for growth and happiness."

There's really nothing nice about a divorce. Sometimes it's the right thing to do for your children. That doesn't make it any easier. The age of your children the reasons surrounding the divorce will play a big role in how your kids will handle it.

Here are a few do's and don'ts when you are discussing divorce with your children.

The Do's

•	If you have children older than 10, they might want to talk to someone other than mom and dad about the divorce. You need to step up to the plate and encourage them to do this. Many children need this outlet in order to trust you again.

•	Right when you decide to separate it's important to sit down and calmly discuss this with your kids. Don't ever tell about it after the fact. Try and keep your emotions under control and you both need to be there for this if that's possible.

•	Sit down and figure out what you are going to say. If you need a counselor for this, make sure you get one. This is huge for your children but it's really not the end of the world.

•	Make sure you address the divorce in an age-appropriate manner, so your children will understand what you are saying. Never tell them the hurtful facts. Try and sugar coat it if you will and definitely don't try and throw one another under the bus. No matter how hurt you might be, that's not something your kids should have to live with.

•	Be as honest as you can but don't give them too much information. The less they know the better, particularly if they are under the age of 10.

•	You don't want to discourage your children from relationships. That said, it's important that you explain to them that sometimes people change and they grow apart. When this happens it's best that instead of fighting, you both move on. Remind them that living apart from each other doesn't have to be a bad thing.

- No matter what, remind your kids that even though the two of you aren't going to be together, that both of you love them very much.

- Please make sure you tell your children over and over again that the divorce is adult stuff and it has nothing to do with them. Often children will think of one instance where they ticked you off and they may try and blame themselves for breaking up mom and dad. Make sure that doesn't happen.

- Let your kids get upset or sad if they want to. Listen to what they have to say and be there for them in a positive manner.

- Do your best to make sure you keep their routine on track. Tell them you will make sure very little changes in their daily life. They need to hear that from you and then you need to show them. That's going to take both of you to make sure that happens.

- Make sure, no matter how much it hurts, that your kids know it's perfectly fine to spend time with your ex and not with you. Parent loyalty comes into the picture here and you've got to reassure your kids that you are okay with them deciding who they want to spend their time with. Honestly, I struggled a little with this one because I wanted them all to myself. Eventually, I got over it and realized they need their father just as much as me, aside from our differences.

- Take action to go to counseling with our ex and with your children. It's very important that your kids have professional guidance through this often traumatic process. This is something I screwed up on and never did.

Ten years after the fact I found out my daughter kept everything bottled up inside and it's been eating her inside out. Get the counseling asap cuz it can't hurt.

The Don'ts

•	Never make fake promises to your kids. That's only going to wind up causing undue stress and distrust.

•	This is a tough one but you need to be on your best behavior and not talk crap about your ex. That's just too easy to do but it's seriously detrimental to your kids.

•	Don't lie to your children and yourself and pretend like nothing is going to change. Everything is going to be different but that doesn't have to be a negative thing. Make sure they understand different doesn't need to be a bad thing.

•	Never make your kids choose a side or give the ammunition to pit one parent against another. They need to understand you both love them equally and respect their feelings always.

•	Don't put your children in the middle of it by using them to get dirt on your ex and what he's doing. If you try to do this you are just putting more conflict into your relationship.

•	Please don't use your kids to relay the message. If you need to talk to your ex about something you need to talk to them, not through the kids. Take the weight off of their shoulders.

•   Don't ever tell your children that their father doesn't love them anymore. No matter how hurt you are, a child needs to believe and know they are loved by BOTH parents equally.

•   Never act in a negative way about your ex so that your kids will see these nonverbal cues. All that's doing is hurting your kids, so just don't do it.

There really is nothing good about divorce when it comes to children. I grew up with a mom and a dad that supported and loved each other no matter what. I was lucky. My children only knew that for a short time and the details of the reasons why I left I would rather keep to myself than to take faith away from the belief they have in their dad.

Does that make sense?

Bottom line is, try to keep this as simple as you can regardless of the circumstances. Your children didn't ask to be born and it's not their fault you aren't still with your ex. Leave the details out, keep it short and sweet, and most of all make sure you are both understanding and supportive.

Your kids need to understand they are loved and they don't need to choose sides under pressure.

You are a great single mom. Show your kids this.

Chapter Eighteen

Mental Health Issues Single Moms Tackle

"I know I'm the only one that can change my life for the better. Nobody else is going to do it for me." CAW

Just think about it for a second, imagine you were suddenly divorced or separated and had to take care of three children, you only earned $30,000 a year, felt your friends and family were drifting away, and consistently felt judged about your parenting style, regardless of how well you're handling it.

Lucky you, welcome to the life of a single mom.

There's no doubt, being a single mom is physically and emotionally demanding. Often being a single mom takes a huge toll on your mental health.

Every day single moms step up to the plate to care for their children. It's too bad many moms don't like to ask for help and many times don't think they need it. For me, life stresses started piling up and started to create mental health issues.

I went through mild bouts of depression and anxiety. Many women struggle silently with other conditions like PTSD. This can lead to self-medicating with drugs, alcohol, or perhaps prescription drugs.

Let's have a look at some common mental health issues single moms struggle with, and perhaps I can inspire you to call a spade and spade and get professional help if you are suffering.

Mental Health Challenge One - Lack Of Solid Sleep

It's safe to say that single moms hardly ever get adequate sleep. For me, it was because the only time I felt I could get things done was when my children were sleeping.

Sleep when the baby sleeps just didn't work for me at the time.

There was always dishes, cleaning, laundry, and so many other household tasks on my list of chores, I actually felt guilty if I went to bed too early when the kids were sleeping. Not getting enough sleep is the volatile platform for many other single mother challenges.

Mental Health Challenge Two - Not Taking Care Of Yourself

Like me, many single moms are too focused on their children to take care of themselves effectively. Lots of single moms can't even find the time or energy for exercise or going to get their nails done.

Everyone deserves a pick me up now and again. Single moms that make the time to take care of themselves are going to be able to better cope with the real challenges of being a single parent.

I used exercise as a way to shift my brain into positive gear. Most days I didn't get as much in as I wanted to but even 15-20 minutes made a huge difference in strengthening my mental health.

Mental Health Challenge Three - Not Being Financially Stable

Often in a divorce, one party, often the mom, winds up trying to live with money stress. Working for minimum wage while affording daycare makes moms feel like they are working for nothing and always coming up short when it comes to paying the bills.

It makes sense that not having any money in the bank is linked directly to anxiety and depression.

I always seemed to be struggling with money. There was enough to get by but not enough to be comfortable and not worry about whether or not my phone or the hydro was going to get shut off.

Mental Health Challenge Four - Little To No Support Systems

It doesn't matter whether by choice or circumstance that a woman winds up being a single mom, more often than not many of her friends disappear when she really needs them. In some cases, friends will choose sides and feel weird being the friend they used to be to you.

Often single moms wind up becoming disconnected with their community and that just leads to that helpless empty feeling of being totally alone.

I tried to keep my balance but it seemed pretty much impossible trying to take care of everything all by myself. There was just no time for me to get out there and stay connected with my friends and family. That's what it felt like anyway.

Mental Health Challenge Five - Ex Drama

Sadly, many divorces end with couple conflict and this certainly takes a toll on a single mother. Lots of moms are forced to face bullying, manipulation, and not abiding by the divorce agreement. All of which are huge stressors to deal with on top of everything else.

For me, there wasn't much of that going on. It's so important for you to seek help if you are having conflicts with your ex.

Mental Health Challenge Six - The Constant Feeling Of Being Judged

You can't get away from the assumed stereotypes of being a single mother. It's stressful not knowing when these judgments will hit you in the face. It could be a family member, other parents, or perhaps a teacher.

These negative assumptions about your parenting skills are unfair.

Nobody should judge anyone else unless they are walking in their shoes.

Mental Health Challenge Seven - Abuse

Truth—The rate of domestic abuse in our society is sickening. Many single mothers are trying to escape abusive relationships. These women are brave to leave their relationship, but they need to understand they have been traumatized psychologically.

For me, that hurt more than the physical. I was abused by my ex-husband but I have experienced abuse.

I never got the help I needed. Even if the abuse you suffered from is in the past, it's important that you take the time to seek professional help. You are not alone.

Mental Health Challenge Eight - Kids With Special Needs

Studies show that families that have children with special needs are more likely to divorce than the general population. And because it's normally the moms that get custody of the children, they wind up taking on this stressful role.

For any single moms that have been challenged with one or more of these mental health issues, here are a few take action steps to help you regain control of your well-being:

•	Ask For Help—The strongest people ask for help when they need it. You are not weak or a failure because you ask for help.

•	Take Care Of You—If you don't take care of yourself, who's going to take care of your children? This is essential and it doesn't have to break the bank.

•	Hook Up With Other Single Moms—Having a strong support system in place is going to make your job as a single mom a heck of a lot easier. Being able to relate with other single moms on a day-to-day basis will make you stronger.

•	Create Your Network—It's important to build yourself a network of family, friends, and acquaintances. You need to make sure your network is there when you need them most.

•	Get Professional Help: Nobody can do this alone. Getting counseling can literally change your quality of life for the better. You don't have to try and do it all and it's crazy to think you should. I hope you can learn from my mistakes.

You deserve to smile from the inside out, that's my belief.

Chapter Nineteen

Inspirational Quotes

I'm a firm believer in gaining inspiration from uplifting quotes. I've written my own quotes for many years and hope you can use my thoughts and beliefs to help make your day more positive, your struggles less stressful.

"The most amazing things in life can't be seen or touched - they're only felt by your heart."

Reflection - We live in a world that moves so fast, where everyone seems to always want more. When it's all said and done you will figure out the most important things in life, things that can't be taken, are felt in your heart.

"The best way you can prepare yourself for tomorrow is to take positive action to do your best today."

Reflection - Nobody knows what's going to happen tomorrow. Life can be taken in the blink of an eye and we need to remember that. If you want to have an amazing tomorrow you need to focus on the positive and accept you are doing your best today.

"If you want to succeed, to inspire others, put all of your mind, heart, and should into everything you do, big or small."

Reflection - I aim to inspire others. Even if I positively touch just one person, I've succeeded. Give everything you do your all and you will both inspire and succeed in all that you do.

"Getting happy isn't something you put off for some time in the future; happiness should be created for the now."

Reflection - So many people, I included, look forward to what might be in the future to find our happiness. I've learned that's not productive, it's actually a little sad. Figure out how to be happy in the now and look forward to more amazing in the future.

"I've tried, but I can't change the direction of the wind, however, I know I can adjust my sails and I will always figure out my destination."

Reflection - So many times in my life I've tried to battle what can't be changed. Silly but it's true. I've learned over the years I can't change the unchangeable but I can control my thoughts and actions to make sure I wind up where I should be.

"Never forget that your health is your most valuable asset. When it's gone I'm afraid it's gone."

Reflection - When you're young you are programmed to believe you are invincible. As the years pass by you realize rather quickly that you aren't. I've learned that taking care of your health; mind, body, and soul, should be your number one priority throughout life. To it sooner rather than later.

"It's truly difficult but it's in your scariest, darkest moments, that you need to stay strong and focus on the beautiful light."

Reflection - Everyone goes through difficult times in life. What you need to remember is that no matter how tough it is, no matter how solid the darkness is around you, there is always hope and you need to focus on the beauty of the light at the end of the tunnel. You have to believe it's there.

"The first thing you need to do is what you have to; then it's time for you to do what's possible; then all of a sudden with positive effort you are doing what you once was impossible."

Reflection - I'm a dreamer and that often gets me into deep trouble. There's always going to be things I have to do, and I will. Next up I try and do what's possible, the things I basically know I can do. In the end, I want to do what I once believed was impossible. I believe that's being truly inspirational. The key is you've got to believe. It's hard but you've gotta do it.

"Everyone has dreams as a child and inspirations. What you need to do is let go of what you thought you wanted in life and accept exactly what's waiting for you. That can be magical too."

Reflection - You grow up innocent, with your mind open to dreaming the impossible. Then I learned fast, what you want and what's going to happen doesn't always align. That just resulted in disappointment. Don't be so hard on yourself. Stay positive and believe in your dreams. However, you are best to let go of what you thought you wanted and accept the beauty in what is. It's still a win.

"There's someone sitting in the shade today simply because someone decided to plant a tree a long time ago."

Reflection - This is a tough one. There are times in life I've learned, where there's someone that just doesn't want you to succeed. It's not hard to hurt another person and block their success. What you need to do is step past this and make sure another person's misery doesn't dictate your success.

"I don't want to just survive in life. I want to thrive with passion, compassion and humor, and perhaps a little style."

Reflection - I'm a survivor but that's not how I want to be defined. I want to push myself forward and show my passion. I want to do this with style and inspiration so I can lead other people down a positive path.

"There are always going to be clouds in my life. I'm not looking to carry the rain or bring on the storms, I just want to add color to me and make my sunset beautiful."

Reflection - Life is full of ups and downs, that's the reality. Nobody wants to bring darkness, I certainly don't. I want to bring the positive with me and hopefully, it always helps to brighten or inspire someone else.

"Motivation is alive when you are working on things that hold meaning for you."

Reflection - It's not always easy to get motivated. For me, I've learned to use my mind to push me forward to get things done. I've made a habit of exercising to get my positive thinking flowing and my energy up, then I have the power and want to get motivated.

Chapter Twenty

Acceptance Quotes

"When you can't find a solution to an issue or problem, it's likely a problem that shouldn't be solved. But more likely a truth that needs to just be accepted."

My Reflection...Sometimes in life, I want so badly to figure something out that is beyond my control or that simply can't be changed. And no matter how hard I try I just spin my wheels and create my own stress and disbelief in me. It's better sometimes to just accept the truth and let it be.

"At some point in life you've just got to let go of what you so badly wanted to believe should happen and embrace and live in the moment of what is happening."

My Reflection...There have been times in my life where I really wanted to believe something so badly it hurt. More often than not the moment never happened. I would have been better to tune into the "now" or "real" moment and never mind the rest. Sometimes my imagination gets away on me.

"The things in life you can't control are telling you to just let go."

My Reflection...Sometimes it just sucks when you don't have control over something you so desperately want. Rather than live in the unknown and hope it's often better just to let go and let nature take its course. If it was meant to be then it was meant to be.

"You need to first love who you are and if you're going to do that you can't hate the experiences that have shaped you; good, bad, and not so good."

My Reflection...I'm still working on this one; loving myself. But I know when I fall in love with me I will better accept some of the tough life experiences I have faced. That's just the way it works.

"The most precious gift you can give anyone is permission to feel safe in their own skin. To feel supported, loved and worthy of who they are. To feel like they are enough."

My Reflection...Life is tough. People are often judgmental and mean spirited. When you show someone you love them for who they are and empower them to become happy in who they are on all levels, accepting their insecurities and supporting their inspirations, you become that special someone that's an integral part of building them stronger. It really doesn't get much better than that.

"I believe one of the happiest moments in life is when you discover the courage to simply let go of what you can't change - period."

My Reflection...Think of all the time we spent fretting about what other people think or about things we just can't change. It's easy really crazy. When you find the strength without you to just leave the stuff alone that you can't change, the doors of peace and opportunity open up.

"My belief is people need to be loved and accepted more than they need advice."

My Reflection...I don't know about you but I know that I care about what other people think and it bothers me when I see someone thinking negative about me. More often than not it's not advice I need but rather plain and pure acceptance for who I am. A love unconditional that really does mean everything.

"The whole world is never going to accept you, want, or know how to receive your energy. Learn to be okay with that and move forward positively."

My Reflection...A tough one for me. Not everyone is going to love me. It really doesn't matter the reasons because you'd go crazy trying to figure it out. The best thing to do is to just let it go and move forward open and optimistic and happy in you.

"When you learn to simply accept rather than expect, I can guarantee your life will have a lot fewer disappointments."

My Reflection...Life gets disappointing from time to time. If you adopt the learned mindset of accepting instead of expecting all the time, you are going to create more positive outcomes. It's not as easy as it sounds but definitely doable.

"The only thing that heals everything is acceptance."

My Reflection...I for one know that time doesn't heal all wounds. Sure it may reduce some of the pain but it doesn't always heal. When you are ready to accept you then heal.

"When you finally accept yourself you get rid of the burden of needing me to accept you."

My Reflection...We are hard on ourselves. I know I'm hard on me but I know the more I accept who I am the less I need to stress about proving my worth through other people. That really is a huge stress because I only control me, nobody else.

Chapter Twenty-One

Mistake Quotes

"Please don't believe every mistake is a foolish one."

My Reflection...Sure there will be times in your life where you make a bonehead mistake; that's life. But don't think that every mistake was avoidable or somehow could have been skipped past. Mistakes are essential to learning and growing and moving forward in life. Without mistakes, you'll just exist and that's a tragedy.

"When you choose to learn from your mistakes you aren't wasting your time, you make it worth your while."

My Reflection...It really is a matter of choice or perspective. You will always look at your mistakes as negative and worthless is you don't look to consciously learn from them, regardless of how difficult they are. I try and stop myself for a moment to look at my mistakes and look for ways to learn from them. Otherwise, I'm just left feeling bad for making a stupid mistake. It's a choice.

"One person will hesitate, afraid of making mistakes. The other will get busy making mistakes and create superior."

My Reflection...Do you think successful people in life don't ever make mistakes? If you do you're sorely mistaken because they are the ones who have made the most mistakes of all. The difference is they choose to overcome them, flip them positive, and never quit on their beliefs. Mistakes are an integral part in creating strong, accomplished, and amazing. Better get busy making mistakes if you truly want to uncover your awesome potential.

"It's your experience that allows you to make mistakes and realize when you make one again."

My Reflection...I am the queen of making mistakes and thankfully I know when I make them, at least eventually I figure it out. I'll admit you do have a problem if you don't know when you muck up.

"A life not filled with mistakes is a wasted life; nothing learned, nothing gained."

My Reflection...There are some people that are afraid to try things because they don't want to screw up. We all have our moments but for the most part I'm okay with mistakes, just means I'm learning what not to do. That may seem a little whacky to you but at least I'm not sitting on my butt twiddling my thumbs wondering what next.

"Your mistakes are a portal to the land of opportunity."

My Reflection...As hard as this sounds it really is a matter of positive mind power. If you learn to look at your mistakes or life missteps as an opportunity, then you don't feel like such a dork when you screw up and you aren't stopping yourself from taking life risks...if that makes sense?

"You have no freedom if you don't accept and understand the importance of making mistakes."

My Reflection...Life is give and take and if you don't recognize and more importantly accept the fact you are going to need to make mistakes to move forward positively in life, to find your true potential, then what sort of life are you really living? You certainly aren't living so you can be free. Freedom of choice includes making mistakes - end of story.

"If you don't make mistakes you will never know what you need to improve and that's just sad."

My Reflection...Once again I'm very seasoned in making mistakes. I try and look at my screw-ups as a door of opportunity to make myself better. It doesn't always work but for the most part, it does and I'll keep on trying.

"Success and action are interconnected. People who are successful make mistakes and keep on moving. They never quit."

My Reflection...If you don't ever take action you can never move forward and be successful. And if you don't make mistakes you are never taking action and my belief is you are missing out. Don't let the fear of making a mistake stop you from taking action in life. That would just be sad.

Chapter Twenty-Two

Overcoming Quotes

"When you hit rock bottom in life, use this to create your foundation for your fabulous life."

My Reflection...There comes a time when the world will run you over. It's safe to say that happens to everyone. It sucks. I'm not there right now but I'm definitely not in the place I want to be, so I get it. It's likely learned from childhood but my forced mentality here is to remind myself consciously that I can really only go up from here. This means I'm still kicking and I'm at the bottom, so anything else that's going to happen has got to be better, moving from the darkness and into at least the shade, preferably the light. Gain strength in your darkest moments to never lose sight of the light and use this to pull yourself out of your rut so you can climb your mountain. Positive mind power is energy.

"It's true the world is loaded with suffering, but don't forget the abundance of overcoming it."

My Reflection...To me, it's about perspective and it's just too easy to get lulled into the negative zone, which really doesn't help anything. I acknowledge so crappy stuff around be because it is real, but I choose to focus on the greater gain from it. Where people beat the odds and create something amazing. It's better than sitting with dark thoughts in my brain. That's one way I manifest my positive energy.

"Real-life success defined is the ability to overcome the fear of being unsuccessful."

My Reflection...Everyone is afraid of something. For me it's stepping outside of what I know to take a stab and something new, seeing if I can actually do it. I know the thought of failing can deter me from even trying. But I try to remind myself if I don't ever take that step I will never change and I won't ever know what real success is. I don't ever want that so I use that thought to find the courage to beat my fears. Scary but worth it.

"By learning to accept what has happened you have taken the first step to overcome the consequences of any misfortune suffered."

My Reflection...We all have had crappy things happen to us. Sometimes those negative thoughts stick in my head and try and overtake me, steal my happiness. When you choose to not be defeated by the wrongs in your life you gain power and strength. This is where you show the world who you really are and that you aren't going to let anyone or anything take away from you. I choose to be happy and I choose to push through the negatives in my life and focus on the positive. This doesn't mean the bad things never happened, it just means I program my brain to make sure I don't lose because life happens. It really is a choice.

"I'm a huge believer in achieving and overcoming and taking action to do things instead of simply making excuses and feeling sorry for yourself."

My Reflection...Excuses are easy. Stepping up to the plate and overcoming your life challenges and fears are not. When you decide to mentally take control and push through issues to achieve your goals, you're heading in the right direction. Put in the effort if you want results. If you want positive change you've simply got to take action.

"First you need to be smart and be aware of your fear. Success comes when you figure out how to overcome your fear."

My Reflection...Awareness for me is the toughest part. Facing your fears is the first step and only route to conquering. Yet many of us, I included, would rather just live with our fears than find the courage to face them and deal with them. The unknown is a scary place. The only way you can truly be successful is if you take the steps you need to that drive you right past your fears. Not easy but you're worth it.

"Life is all about obstacles. When you learn to overcome your obstacles you find satisfaction and purpose."

My Reflection...Life is loaded with challenges, obstacles good and bad that you've got to work through in order to find your purpose and ultimately reach your goals. Your purpose can only be found if you are willing to step outside your comfort zone and face your life challenges. Don't think about it...just do it.

"Keeping busy with fresh activity and newness is the only route to overcoming adversity."

My Reflection...To move forward in life is to grow and if you are looking to break through your self-set barriers the easiest route to do this is by getting active and experiencing new. This is only going to open doors of opportunity and ensure you have the power to move forward positively. Information is knowledge and knowledge is power, never forget it.

"Life will always have obstacles. Your key to happiness is learning how to open your mind and believe in yourself to find your happiness."

My Reflection...If you truly want to be happy inside-out you've got to understand and accept you will have roadblocks along the way. Make a point of consciously believing in yourself and pushing yourself past the barriers in front of you because fabulous really is just over the next hill. Believe it.

"The greater the obstacle the more spectacular the reward of overcoming it."

My Reflection...Life is hard and sometimes we get a challenge in front of us that just seems impossible to overtake. The truth...the bigger the obstacle the greater the reward. Program your brain to think this way and amazing will begin unfolding and just never stop. That's my belief.

Chapter Twenty-Three

Believe Quotes

Dreams

"Never stop dreaming. Understand to reach your goals requires belief in you, determination, perseverance, vision, and faith. When you believe anything is possible."

Mirror

"You only hear what you want to hear; you only see what you choose to see. Your belief system is simply a mirror that shows you what you truly believe."

Mindpower

"I believe in the power of positive energy, that your positive thinking and belief helps you create your great. My belief."

Success

"You aren't born into success. It's created with pure untainted belief."

Passion

"Passionate belief is the key to succeeding personally and in business. Why should anyone be proud of what you are doing if you aren't? Just saying…"

Foundation

"By knowing who you are and believing in yourself no matter what, well that's your stepping stone to greatness."

Attitude

"Having a positive attitude, belief and commitment are vital to success. Doesn't matter whether you are in business or sports or school; belief matters."

Failure

"Consciously believing everything is going to be just fine means you get your butt to work because failing isn't even in your brain."

Change

"Making real change is tough. You need to be grounded, know who you are, believe in yourself and understand what you can really do; you can make a difference."

Chapter Twenty-Four

Happiness Quotes

"Happiness is mastering the art of never holding your mind to the memory of any unpleasant occurrence that has passed...Moving forward positively."

"If you are going to be truly happy you can't be too concerned with the thoughts of other people."

"When I want simple happiness for an hour - I take a nap."

"True moments of happiness take us by surprise. I don't seize these moments...they sneak up and seize me...magical."

"It's not who you are, what you have, where you are, or what you are doing that makes you happy; it's what you are thinking about."

"The direct route to happiness is to stop worrying about the oodles of things in life you can't control, the power of your will."

"There are times it's your smile that creates happiness, and other times it's happiness that creates your beautiful smile."

"Real love is when the happiness of another is essential to yours."

"The happy people of the world plan to take action, they never plan results."

"When what you are thinking, saying, and doing, are within the same beat, that's happiness."

"Some people create happiness wherever they go; others suck it up but never create it."

"I smile knowing nobody has been "uncheered" with a balloon.

"Newsflash...Your measure of success isn't the key to your happiness. It's your happiness that will trigger your success. Yes, they work hand in hand but don't kid yourself, one certainly leads the other."

"The controllable cause of unhappiness is these false beliefs rattling around in your head; these beliefs are often so common and widespread you never think to question them."

"Pinky swear promise me you will never forget happiness comes from your action."

"Sure there will be doors of happiness that will close on you. Stop yourself from focusing on the freakin closed door or you will miss that magical doors opening for you."

"Choose to laugh at life not frown over it."

"I believe people find it difficult to be happy because they seem to view the past as better than it was, the now as worse than it really is, and the future of indecision as the scary unknown. How about looking at it as a magical opportunity."

"The truth to me is you can almost always enjoy something if you decide you are going to find happiness in it...it really is a choice."

"When you accept yourself you will find happiness...my belief."

"The key to happiness is not doing what you like all the time, rather it's liking what you do."

"There are many people out there that choose to make sure they are miserable instead of risking the chance to be happy."

"Unhappy people find comfort in the misfortunes of others...super sad."

"Caution comes in all shapes and forms, be careful, caution in love is most fatal to happiness."

"I believe the most beautiful people in the world know defeat, have suffered, know about struggling, have experienced loss, and have always found a way out of the darkness - no excuses. These people have an appreciation, sensitivity, and understanding of life that overloads them with compassion, empathy, gentleness, and genuine loving concern. It's true, beautiful people inside-out don't just happen."

"There's more happiness to be had when you are making other people happy. You should put more thought into all the happiness you have to give...just saying."

Chapter Twenty-Five

Living Life To The Fullest Quotes

"When all is said and done, you'll only regret the chances you decided not to take."

"Your life is an experiment. The more experiments you choose to take the better."

"Look at your life as a game, play it; Your life is a challenge, Meet it without reserve; Your life is an open book opportunity, Grab hold and make the most of it."

"If you try and obey all the rules, you're going to skip right past all the fun in life."

"Wanna hear something sad? You should have, you could have, and you might have."

"When you're gone, the only thing that's going to matter is the time between the two dates. Make the most of it."

"Twenty-five years from now you are going to be much more disappointed in the things you didn't do, not the things you did."

"Give thanks for your yesterdays, live for the moment, and dream of tomorrow."

"Don't you think it's about time you let go of the handrails? — Let go...give in and live with excitement and passion every day."

"Stay strong and let the positive forces around take hold. In the past, when I've fallen short, it's always been because I let the fear of failure derail me, not because I tried and screwed up."

"If you want to get the most out of life, step up to the plate and view it as an amazing adventure."

"A few questions you should ask yourself every day: "What's good in your life? And "What needs to be changed?"

"Cause and effect work hand in hand. If your life has no cause it can't have any effect either."

"There is one ultimate success, that's to live your life the way you want to."

"Never put things off for another day. Create your memories today and celebrate what you can have in the now."

"The only limitations your life has, are the ones you create."

"Think about your life as a nice big canvas. Throw as much paint on it as you can."

"Never be afraid your life might end. Be afraid that it might never really begin."

"As far as I know you only live once. If you open your mind to opportunity and do it right, once is more than enough."

"It would have been nice if someone told me when I was born that I was dying. Then I may have lived every minute of every day and never let my inhibitions get in the way of

what could have been. Do what you want to do right now. There might not be too many tomorrows."

"You might need to be reminded that the purpose of your life is to live it to the fullest. Reach out without fear and taste the world. When you leave your fears on the side your life will be richer and fuller."

"Don't be fooled. It's not the number of years in your life that matters. It's the life in your years that says it all."

"If you really want to smile, don't focus on the past, don't fret about the future, tune in on living fully, right now in the present."

"If you are set to overcome the anxiety of life, live in the now, live and breath in this moment."

"Being 'single" enables you to live your life on your own terms without apology."

"It's possible I'm not going anywhere in life, but wow, what a ride."

"Take action to seize each day, then release it."

"It's vital to live in each moment...just don't be controlled by the moment or the people who are in it."

"If you happen to be struggling today, don't forget that every life is worth living and believe your amazing is just around the corner. You are loved, you are important, and never ever forget there will always be hope, a light at the end of the dark tunnel."

"Being creative isn't just about thinking outside the box, it's always about living there."

"Let each new day be your own new beginning; learn, grow, admire, love. Get excited about all the possibilities at your fingertips."

"Mindfulness isn't about entering another planet. It's all about making you amazing at what you do. It's simply restoring your direct like to the ultimate source of life."

"It really doesn't matter what people tell you because your thoughts, feelings, and words can and will change the world if you believe and don't quit."

"There's no doubt, with determination, perseverance, and the right support, you can achieve anything."

"Life is full of all sorts of challenging twists and turns. All you need to do is hold on tight and take flight."

"You're more than enough exactly as you are. Don't you dare change a thing."

"I choose to not just exist. My mission is to not just survive day to day, I want to thrive."

Take action to create your future now, and focus on making your dreams reality tomorrow."

"If you open your mind, you'll let life change in a positive way very fast."

"There's no doubt in my mind, you get what you give in life."

"It's very important to do the things in life you believe you can't do."

"Understand that nothing is impossible. Look at the word, it say's "I'm possible."

"For me, I've found that happiness often slips in through the door when you didn't realize you left it open."

"You should always face toward the sun so the shadows are always behind you."

"You are never too old to try something new, set a new goal, or capture a new dream."

"Life is just like riding a bike. If you want to keep your balance you just can't stop, you've got to keep on moving."

"It's important that you stay as close as you can to the things that make you happy you're alive."

"What matters in life isn't where you came from. It's where you are headed that counts."

"I try to be a magical rainbow in someone else's cloud."

"You've got to make your happy, it's not going to suddenly find you."

"A day is wasted if it's not full of laughs."

"If I'm unable to do great things that's okay. I choose to do the small things in an awesome way."

Having a plan isn't always the right choice. There are times when you just need to breathe, believe, trust, let go, and just wait and see what happens."

"The sad news is that time flies. The great news is that you get to be the pilot."

"There are going to be times where you never really know the value of a moment, not until it's a fast memory."

"When you focus on having only good thoughts, the will ultimately shine out of your face like beautiful sunbeams, and you will always look amazing. It comes from the inside out."

"It's truly the simple that creates the amazing."

"The only thing you need is the plan, a road map, and the courage and determination to push forward to your final destination."

"There's no doubt, the glow of one warm thought is worth more than anything money could buy."

"When you believe in yourself you can risk curiosity, you can wonder with spontaneous delight. You can take control and experience all that your human spirit will allow."

Chapter Twenty-Six

Passion Quotes

"How are you supposed to rely on your eyes if your imagination is completely out of focus."

"You can't find passion without risk - they walk hand in hand. Don't settle for a life less than what you are capable of living - promise me."

"Passion is energy. Concentrate on that power, the energy that excites you internally. Take your passion and run with it. Never walk past it."

"If you want to feel your passion in your veins you've got to take action on it."

"Passion is one of those things in life that you can't fake."

"Tell your story with passion or don't tell it."

"If you think there's something out there you should be doing, something that draws you to it, then you need to stop wishing and find the courage to take action and do it - end of story."

"Your soul only knows what it knows and it can only be true to its own desires. To master its passion it must abandon itself."

"Don't you dare give up, don't ever."

"It's true, you can become successful at almost anything that you are enthusiastic about."

"To me, courage is skipping from failure to failure without losing your spark."

"Ask yourself what makes you come alive, then go do it. What our world needs is people that have come alive."

"Passion and purpose walk hand in hand. When you find your purpose you will uncover your passion - they are collectively exhaustive."

"It's passion that elevates you and takes you to greater things."

"Let your passion become your purpose. Do this and one day your passion will become your profession."

"Be fearless when you're chasing what sets your soul on fire."

"Passion. Enable power to your calling. Focus intently into your heart's beat. Breathe it. Live it. Be it."

Chapter Twenty-Seven

Positive Change Quotes

"All positive change starts with a clear decision to either quit doing something or to start."

"I believe with each positive change you make in your life you'll change something else for the better - chain reaction - magical."

"You'll discover your new direction in the waves of change."

"Please never be scared of change because that's where you will be gifted in your new direction."

"If you are trying to change the direction of the wine, strop, just adjust your sails."

"Dear Past, I appreciate all the tough life lessons. Dear Future, I'm finally ready."

"The tip-top secret of change is to tune all your positive energy not into fighting the past, just use it to create and build NEW."

"Promise me you will never be scared of change. Sure you will lose some good things but that's how you create better."

"Progress forward can't happen without change. And if you can't change your thinking you're never going to change anything."

"It's time to stop expecting other people to take action first, you need to be the one that creates positive change."

"When you commit to change how you look at things, I pinky-swear promise those things you focus on will change."

"Truth...Chance doesn't make your life better, change does."

"It's simple, if you really don't like something change it; and if it's something you can't change, you need to change the way you think about it."

"My belief is when you are set to make positive changes in your life you'll attract everything you need to succeed."

"If you want to change your life you've got to change your priorities."

"Is change easy? Nope. Is it worth it? Absolutely."

"Dream a little. Make a wish. Don't be afraid to take a chance. Make your change."

"IF you are re-reading your last chapter in your life there's' no way you can start another one."

"Change is a part of life that can't be stopped, it's not always controllable. But what you can control is how you react, manage, and work to make change positive."

Chapter Twenty-Eight

Fear Quotes

"Fear is simply your brain signaling to you there's something VIP for you to tackle and overcome."

"The truth is...Fear is completely temporary. Your regrets could last forever."

"Your fears are NOT your limitations, not ever."

"In truth fear is an adventure-crushing, idea-bashing, success-suffocating interference factor created by YOURS truly."

"Did you know that fear kills far more dreams than actual failure will?"

"Fear...It's a choice...Choose to forget it all and run far and far...OR...Rise to the challenge and face it all."

"Believe any and all you ever wanted is just on the other side of fear."

"Fear is manifested in YOUR mind. It's a creation of your thoughts. Danger, on the other hand, is real, however, your fear is CHOICE."

"FEAR is...False Evidence Appearing Real."

"The things you fear most are exactly what you need to do."

"You need to figure out that you want it much more than you are afraid of it."

"I have STRENGTH...

Because I accept my weaknesses.

I have BEAUTY...

Because I know my flaws.

I am chosen FEARLESS...

Because I've learned the difference between real and fake.

I am WISE...

Because I learn and grow from my life screw-ups.

I choose to LOVE...

Because hate makes me cry.

I choose to SMILE...

Because frowning isn't inspirational."

"It's your biggest fear that transports your most amazing feat of growth."

"Each day you emerge stronger than you were yesterday. Choose to face your fears and dry your tears."

"If you want to succeed you need to one in on your conscious thoughts and not the things you worry and fear.

"Unfortunately many of us are not living our dreams because we let our fears dictate our path."

"Let your BELIEF outshine your fears."

"The only thing that can kill your dreams is self-created FEAR."

Know the fear of suffering is always much worse than the suffering itself."

"My courage rises when fear attempts to knock me down flat."

"Afraid is what you might be feeling and Courageous is what you are doing."

"When you surrender to your fears you kill the communication with your heart."

"Most men will do whatever it takes to avoid fear instead of achieving what they desire."

"When you choose to understand more you naturally fear less."

"Without fear, there is no fear there is no courage."

"When you overcome your fears you have found freedom."

"If you want to poison fear just laugh."

"Enter the cave you fear because it holds the treasure you're searching for."

Take action to do what you are afraid of."

"Our world is beautiful and awful things will happen. Have no fear. Don't be paralyzed by it."

"It's okay to have fears, what's critical is how you choose to face them."

"I would much rather die with a smile than fret about everything in fear."

"Don't be afraid of failing. Be afraid of not aiming high enough."

"If you allow your mind to focus too much on your fears you've already lost."

"Fear will manipulate you. It has the sneaky power to trick you into existing, living a ho-hum boring life."

"A courageous person feels fear, doesn't get rid of it but takes action to face fear and win."

"Don't base your decisions on fear and what may or may not happen."

"Most people are terrified of what they know coming to an end."

"The smartest route for you to deal with fear is straight up, head-on, just face it."

"If you allow your mind to fear demons they will surround you and eat you up whole."

"Don't allow fear to paralyze you, just accept it and deal with it head-on."

"Does it really matter if what you are scared off is real or a figment of an overactive imagination?"

"I am not afraid of life or death, I'm terrified of waking up one day to realize I forgot to live."

"The only way your fear survives is because of YOU."

"I'm motivated when I'm overcoming my life challenges and surpass the hurdles and obstacles life throws my way. No doubt there will always be oodles out there to motivate and inspire me."

Never Give Up Quotes...

"The way I learn and grow is to face my life obstacles and commit to overcoming them. That's when the magic just begins."

"When you learn how to believe in you, overcoming gets easier."

"Learning how to overcome adversity is essential for love. It helps you realize it's worth a few uphill climbs."

"I believe sports is a metaphor for achieving and overcoming against the odds. A great athlete knows how to lead by example and rise to the challenge - no excuses."

"There is no feeling like overcoming something that truly scares you. Inspiring and powerful."

"Don't try and do everything yourself. Ask the experts. Let people help. Gather the information you need and then just do it."

"I am so much more than my scars."

"Don't make the mistake of trusting someone that claims they really don't give a crap what people think of them. Instead of overcoming obstacles they either pretend they don't exist or make excuses. You are better than that."

"People that don't know how to suffer are worse off than you might believe. Sometimes the only "right" thing you can do in life is to suffer and deal with it until you have the mental power to overcome it and find a better day."

"Sometimes you've got to say "no" in life. Mainly because you need your downtime so you don't look like a jerk because you have nothing left to give. And battling the appetite that comes with the stress of overcommitment is the worst. Keep that part to yourself. Just say "no" and smile and you will be better for it."

"Your perception is everything. Take your limitations and turn them into a golden opportunity. Take your opportunity and transform it into a huge adventure by allowing yourself to dream big."

"Truth...if you expect your life to be simple, your challenges will be overwhelming. If you understand life will be challenging, your life will be easier."

"If you can think it you can overcome it, you CAN overcome any problem."

"There are fish that love swimming upstream and there are some people empowered by overcoming challenges."

"There are people that want and need a superhero to take care of them. I am my own superhero. I just need me, my strengths and secured passions deep in to be overcome any and all obstacles in life. I believe in me."

"Shifting forward in life doesn't mean you get to avoid the pain, instead look past the clouds for a new day despite the raindrops."

"Life seems to keep on throwing rocks at me and I just keep on turning them into sparkly diamonds."

"Look for opportunity hidden in crisis. Dwelling on the pain will suck the life out of you."

"Life has beat the hell out of me many times. But I still choose to love life, same as the flowers loving the sunshine."

Chapter Twenty-Nine

Risk Quotes

"Sure, a boat is certainly safe at the port but that isn't what boats are for."

"When you risk nothing you are really risking everything."

"Do you believe love is a risk? So what if it just doesn't work? The flip side..what if it does?"

"You will accomplish nothing extraordinary without risking."

"Fabulous accomplishments are forever interconnected with big risk."

"The largest risk you will ever have is the one you choose not to take."

"Newsflash...Life is risk and without it, you are sadly selling yourself short."

"IF you ever stumble across that person that makes your heart flutter, stop doubting and take the risk."

"VIP - Take Risks - When you win, you'll be smiling and if you lose, you'll be wise."

"It's the people that choose to risk going too far that will discover how far you can freely go."

"Insanity and Risk...Don't repeat the same action and expect different results. Take a risk. Change your actions - Risk getting a different result."

"If someone offers you their sea in their spacecraft, don't ask where it is! Get on and go for it!"

"You're not going to find a pearl onshore. If you want one you'll have to muster up the courage to dive for it."

"If you feel like you're in control of your life you better take action to speed it up a few notches."

"The only risk in life you need to avoid like the plague is the risk of doing nothing."

"You better step out on the branch where the fruit is."

Understand this...the universe doesn't have any restrictions. It's YOU that places limitations on the universe with your self-created limitations."

"If you are truly looking to succeed, you much create a deep-down desire to rise far above your fear of failure."

"You don't know when your time is up. Better not waste it trying to live for everyone else."

"If you are afraid of risking the peculiar you'll simply have to accept plain old ordinary - so sad."

"There's only one path to avoid being criticized and that's to say nothing, do nothing, and be nothing."

"If you aren't searching to build your dreams, another person is going to rent you to help build theirs - scary."

"Don't EVER accept someone else's thoughts of happiness for you. There is no 'one size fits all' when it comes to YOUR happiness - You decide."

"Don't pay attention to realistic. Choose to go with passion first."

"Just jump, the net WILL appear."

"Ignore the Yahoos that say it can't be done - think big."

"Taking risks is all about succeeding and failing; mutually exclusive; collectively exhaustive; both equally vital."

"When I choose to let go of what I am, I open the magical door to what I WILL be."

"Don't be too skittish about your actions. Your life is an experiment. And the more experiments you have the better."

"Don't ever give up on what you could have been. If you want it, go get it."

"The difference between a person that succeeds and fails is courage."

"Every human dies but sadly some don't ever really live... it's choice."

"You really can't live without mucking up, unless you live so cautiously you aren't really living at all, and that means you've failed miserably."

"Never mind about failing. You should be worried about all the opportunities you will miss if you don't even try."

"Step across your intimidating line of fear and your dreams will come true."

"It's unrealistic to think you can have everything you want, you can't. However, you CAN have everything that truly matters to you."

"It's critical you trust your gut. Your mistakes inevitably should be your own to learn and grow from don't you think?"

"The day will come when the risk to sit still in the pain will be more painful than the risk to run up the flipping mountain."

"The question in my brain isn't about who's going to let me in, rather what person is going to try and keep me out."

Final Words

I know single moms can succeed because I've done it, the long way around of course. For me it's all about perspective and accepting that life might not always go the way you dreamed it would. That's not a bad thing.

You are strong.

You have your children.

You have your health.

No matter how difficult it gets there are sunny skies just around the corner. Your kids need you.

I'm strong but I have learned over the years that I can break. I never accepted help. I wouldn't even let myself cry for fear of being seen as weak.

Don't let this happen to you.

Lean on the people you need to. Cry when you need to. Forgive yourself and look forward to the amazing that is around the corner. Do what you need to in order to survive, always keeping your children first. Never drag them through the crap of a nasty divorce. Protect them from that, set your limitations and do your best.

Take care of yourself; give to yourself because you deserve it.

Single women have the toughest job in the world. You should be proud of yourself. Believe in what will be and understand your kids need you to be strong for them.

Most importantly, find your true happy.

One last thing!

I want to give you a **one-in-two-hundred chance** to win a **$200.00 Amazon Gift card** as a thank-you for reading this book.

All I ask is that you give me some feedback, so I can improve this or my next book :)

Your opinion is *super valuable* to me. It will only take a minute of your time to let me know what you like and what you didn't like about this book. The hardest part is deciding how to spend the two hundred dollars! Just follow this link.

http://reviewers.win/singlemoms

www.ingramcontent.com/pod-product-compliance
Lightning Source LLC
Chambersburg PA
CBHW031227250726
48655CB00005B/1840